Praise for Smart Chi: Warrior's Manual to Constitutional Energy Management

I enjoyed this book from beginning to end. It encouraged me physically, it challenged me mentally, and it moved me spiritually. Wherever you want to go, Ark will take you there!

—Maria Abbatantuono
Certified Fitness Trainer / Certified Group Instructor

Outstanding and very original. It's the perfect book for the martial artist that wants to take his/her performance to the next level and get immersed into a more mindful and perhaps a spiritual training. I think any type of athlete could benefit from its guidelines. The yogic approach mixed with martial arts makes it a very unique contribution, special and inspiring.

—Priscilla Ortiz-Plata
RYT 200 (Ashtanga & Vinyasa Flow Instructor)

With an emphasis on treating the whole being, this manual provides a guide for the individual to explore their physical, mental, emotional, and spiritual self and create a harmonious relationship with the universe and the true self. Featured in this work are exercises, techniques and practices, as well as nutritional guidelines, which begin the reader's journey of positive change and encourage the practitioner to delve within to become the best version of themselves.

—Valerie Canela
CPT ACSM,PTA Global Certified Wellness and Health Coach

Smart Chi

Other Works by Arjunacharya Dasa

Transcendental Warrior I
Serving in the Army of Lord Krishna

Transcendental Warrior II
Let the Battle Begin

Transcendental Warrior III
Clearing the Battlefield

Krishna Warrior Fitness Challenge
The Workout of Your Life

Smart Chi

Warrior's Manual to Constitutional Energy Management

By Arjunacharya Dasa

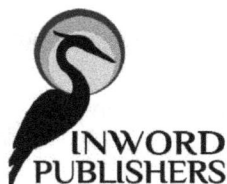

INWORD
PUBLISHERS

For more information, demos and workout videos please visit:
https://www.CompleteWarriorFitness.com
Arjunacharya dasa (Ark Madej)
artofbody@yahoo.com

Cover Artwork: Greg Madej, Steel Soul Productions
Interior Photos: Iguanafoto

Interior Design and Layout: Bhakti-rasa
InwordPublishers.com

Genre: martial arts / self-improvement

Dedication

I dedicate this book to my dear wife, Kasia,
to whom I am always indebted,

and to my sons, Nitai and Nila Madhava, who
always keep me in a state of pleasant alert.

Dedication

Acknowledgments

I offer my sincere gratitude to those who train with me. I continue to learn and improve myself because of the work we do together. We are forever students.

I would like to acknowledge and offer a special thanks to the following individuals for their financial support of the production of Smart Chi, without which I would not have been able to complete this book in a timely manner:

Audree Samuelson, Krishna Adabala, Govinda Dasa, Zdzislaw Madej, Jozefa Madej, Surya Namaskar, the Niekrasz family, Ronald Brandt, David Robison, Eileen Katz, Mr. and Mrs. Micheal Jung, Warriors Jeff and Jen, Kristen Ramsden Oakey, Valerie Kinney, Anonymous donor, Marcin Lech, Cindy Limas, Paul Goldenberg, Phil Kuk, and Danica Dela Fuente.

yad ahankaram ashritya
na yotsya iti manyase
mithyaisha vyavasayas te
prakritis tvam niyokshyati

"If you do not act according to my direction and do not fight, then you will be falsely directed. By your nature, you will have to be engaged in warfare."

Bhagavad-Gita 18.59

shauryam tejo dhritir dakshyam
yuddhe chapy apalayanam
danam ishvara-bhavash cha
kshatram karma svabhava-jam

"Heroism, power, determination, resourcefulness, courage in battle, generosity, and leadership are the natural qualities of work for the *kshatriyas* [warriors]."

Bhagavad-Gita 18.43

Table of Contents

Chapter III – Physical Armor:
Building Blocks for Body and Mind per Body Type 41

Chapter IV – Subtle Armor:
Rediscovering the Secrets of Ancient Masters 60

Chapter V – Spiritual Armor:
Mantras of Ancient Masters

Yogic Mantra – Polishing the Mirror of the Mind
Mantras per Your Constitution
Herbal Supplementation Can Strengthen the Yoga-
    Mantra Practice
Optimum Amount of Tension in the Systems (OATS)

Chapter VI – Warrior Daily Planner

General Strategy for Harmonious Martial Arts
    Training
Training for the Vata
    • Vata-Harmonizing Daily Routine
Training for the Pitta
    • Pitta-Harmonizing Daily Routine
Training for the Kapha
    • Kapha-Harmonizing Daily Routine
Mixed Types
    • Training for Vata-Pittas
    • Training for Vata-Kaphas
    • Training for Pitta-Kaphas
Sample Karate-Based Workout for Vata Constitution
Sample Karate-Based Workout for Pitta Constitution
Sample Karate-Based Workout for Kapha Constitution
Other Workout Routines for Warriors

Preface

In the last fifty years, martial arts in their various forms have transformed and evolved in the West to a point where their practitioners exhibit excellent physical skill. Such level of development no doubt requires a great deal of consistent practice and mental focus. Specifically in the last thirty years, we have seen the rise of mixed martial arts that test the practitioner's combative capabilities to a degree few tournaments ever do.

My own practice of martial arts, mainly under the guidance of Shihan, Master Instructor, in the earlier years, led me to continue my own search for a deep meaning to my martial arts training. As much as I love staying up to date on the MMA today, in staying true to the traditional spirit of martial arts, I must honestly admit that commercialized martial arts tournaments, however real they may be and however accurately they may test one's combative ability, are unnecessarily promoting violence in a world that is already full of it. Many individuals are getting unnecessarily injured or depleted of their own life force prematurely. Those who watch may follow in their footsteps or just become more prone to display violent behavior. This is one of the main triggers for writing this book. As much as it may sound like a cliché these days, I can't restrain myself from quoting the still relevant Taoist sage Lao Tsu:

> *A good soldier is not violent.*
> *A good fighter is not angry.*
> *A good winner is not vengeful.*
> *A good employer is humble.*
> *This is known as the virtue of not striving.*
>
> *This is known as the ability to deal with people.* (68)

Some may say that our society has much more serious problems to solve than unnecessary violence in sports. Sure, but I do not plan on fixing the big problems the world has—I will try to help with what I know I like and am best at. I wish that every individual in society would try to perform their occupations perfectly, trying to help themselves, their family, and society at large. Then, the face of the world would change. On the other hand, if we all do something half-throttle, never becoming the best at what we do, never really caring about the society and the world, nothing will change, and we will just succumb to the social tendencies that will drag us further down into the abyss of lust, anger, and greed.

Looking at our fragile society, it seems that these days we carry around more weapons than ever before, but we experience more fears and attract more violent behavior. People seem to believe that more weapons will give them some level of safety, but they miss the fact that their real armor is the character they develop. It is not about who can climb a higher post and speak louder and more eloquently but about service-oriented action. Martial artists have so much potential to lead the way toward right action (see appendix I for the *Bhagavad-Gita's* recommended way of guiding society). The *Tao Te Ching* hints at that:

> *Why is the sea king of a hundred streams?*
> *Because it lies below them.*
> *Therefore it is the king of a hundred streams.*
>
> *If the sage would guide people, he must serve with humility.*
> *If he would lead them, he must follow behind.*
> *In this way when the sage rules, the people will not feel oppressed.* (66)

Ernest Hemingway wrote that "there is nothing noble in being superior to your fellow man; true nobility is being superior to your former self."

The idea of this book is then to redirect your own combative practice in such a way that you rediscover your true identity and happiness behind the externals of styles, belts, victories, defeats, and teams. Why would you want to do that? Simply because it is the best way you can practice martial arts for the well-being of yourself and society at large, and hence the title of the book is *Smart Chi*. You can certainly expand and channel the harmony achieved through such martial arts practice to encompass all other aspects of life. If you do not desire your own well-being or do not care about society and the world, then this book will still enlighten you in its own way. Want to bet? Let me give you a little peek into what secrets you will find in this one million and eighth book on martial arts.

Discovering your own body type and mental constitution will teach you what to focus on in martial arts training so that you can achieve your maximal potential physically, mentally, and spiritually. Thus, as implied by this work's subtitle, *Warrior's Manual to Constitutional Energy Management*, you will expand the traditional meaning of your skeletal and muscular structure to encompass the psychological, mental factor as well as the factor of pure consciousness (spirit). You will know exactly how to adjust and control your combative practice so that your life force will flow unimpeded as a river flows toward the ocean. You will always have the knowledge to stay clearheaded, and your heart will be purified of all the chaos that got in there knowingly or unknowingly. You will know the meaning of peace. Then you can love and truly help others.

Whatever I share with you in this book is derived from my own experience and the following main sources: Ayurveda (medical science of ancient India), the *Bhagavad-Gita* (ancient scripture on how a warrior should behave), and the *Tao Te Ching* (ancient treatise on how to live in harmony with the universe). It has almost been three decades since the first time I walked into the dojo, and I can say without a doubt that these great texts should be taught in every martial arts school, academy, or institute. If you can find something that will make your martial arts even better, great! I will take a lesson from you.

Another inspiration behind writing this book is writing purely for the art of it and sharing with other fellow practitioners. I have a tinge of desire to express my new thoughts or more-consolidated ideas connected to martial arts practice. If enough of you read this book, I will open up an institute and teach more (the institute is described in chapter VI).

Throughout the book, I will use the following terminology interchangeably:

- Chi—energy, life force, Prana, Ki
- Vata-Pitta—VP
- Vata-Kapha—VK
- Pitta-Kapha— PK
- Individual constitution—body type
- Warrior—martial artist, athlete, fitness enthusiast

Throughout the book, I will attempt to explain three levels of body typing: the physical level (muscles, bones), subtle/psychological level (mind, intelligence), and atma level (spirit, consciousness). The most practical and essential change martial artists can make these days is to align their practices more suitably at the subtle/

psychological level. Once that is made, the other two levels will follow to reveal the most confidential grouping or typing: that according to one's level of consciousness. That is based on an ancient Sanskrit verse from the *Bhagavad-Gita*: "The working senses are superior to dull matter; mind is higher than the senses; intelligence is higher than the mind; and he [the soul] is even higher than the intelligence." (Bg. 3.42) Even though the atma level is the most important aspect of one's being, because it is generally understood very vaguely, I will not focus on it in this book (see my *Transcendental Warrior* book trilogy for the more spiritual approach). Rather, I will explain the physical and psychological body-typing methods and strategies for training.

The above verse is explained by my teacher as follows: "Materially, prescribed duties are duties enjoined according to one's psychological condition, under the spell of the modes of material nature." (Bg. 3.35, purport) It is implied here that your psychological condition should be known to you. Your training coach or instructor should know your mental disposition well enough to prescribe the proper regimen. "Regimen" means not only mere "physical training" but also nutrition, meditation, and general mode of action in daily life. In other words, your combative practice should be undertaken with full understanding of your psychological and physical type. Then there is a very good chance that true spiritual potency will be unleashed from the core of your being.

All glories to Bhaktisiddhanta Sarasvati Thakura the lion educator of this age! (Dec 17, 2016)

Introduction

External Training Approach: Externalization of Modern Martial Arts and Sports

The term "externalization" is used by me to denote a primarily result-oriented, empirically detectable, and measurable progression of a combat or sports athlete. We live in a world that measures our physical characteristics, such as weight, height, reach, and stride, as well as our average and best up-to-date scores in the career and compares us against other warriors or players of opposing teams. To qualify or to make a team, we surely must fulfill certain requirements. For example, we must bench-press our own weight a certain number of times to make a football team, we must have fought a certain number of fights to advance from amateur to professional, we must be able to run a mile under six minutes to join a runner's club—you name it. I am sure you are familiar with the picture I am attempting to describe.

Not only that, but once we have attained the desired status, in order to maintain it, we must protect the status quo by performing according to established standards. For example, we must be winning at least one out of three fights; we must be maintaining our training regimen not to fall off the thin edge of the elite-reserved spot; we must maintain the right weight; we must be studying the strategies of other fighters/opponents to see that we always stay ahead while hunting for newer and better strategies of play.

Finally, should it happen that one lose their cherished spot on the team, most top combatants search for the means to get things back to where they were and are thus oppressed by the desire to re-create the situation that they enjoyed and that cost them so much strife. Some of them, already at the top of their glory or way past their peak years of performance, decide to take a step back and focus on instructing the younger generation.

The modern training and competitive mood of martial arts, which in many aspects of the game resembles an all-out fitness workout, is also monitored strictly with regard to such variables as heart rate, maximum oxygen uptake (VO2), recovery heart rate, speed of various strikes, acceleration of movement, number of punches or kicks delivered, calories expanded during workout, etc. In addition, during the day, the athlete may be strictly supervised by their coaches or by himself/herself for calories burned throughout the day, calories consumed in the day from the right kind of sources, etc.

The whole process of maturation of the warrior, as well as later progressions, is veiled in stress that is born from externalization of one's consciousness or life force. Another descriptive term that may be used here is "fragmentization" of the person. The combat athlete is seen and assessed in terms of the external performance of a multitude of his/her parts rather than as a whole person. Stress is born due to excessive preoccupation with the external environment. Stress creates imbalance in one's body and mind system and sooner or later is the causative factor behind all physical and mental illness.

Internal Training Approach: Three Types of Armor

In direct contrast to the above External Training Approach (ETA) is the Internal Training Approach (ITA), which zeroes in on the proper nourishment and unfolding of the five types of Chi described later in the book. The Supreme Warrior Krishna instructs warrior Arjuna on the battlefield about this balanced approach: "He who is regulated in his habits of eating, sleeping, recreation, and work can mitigate all material pains by practicing the yoga system." (Bg. 6.17) Whether we perform martial arts for recreation or our full-time occupation, it is recommended that we adjust our nutrition and sleeping patterns, and saturate martial arts with a suitable yoga practice.

The first level of training is the training of the physical body, the physical armor, via combative, fitness-oriented, or yoga-oriented movements. The second level of training is the exercise of the subtle armor, which consists of mind, intelligence, and our ego. That is accomplished by specific and proper breathing methods conducted during or separate from one's physical training. This subtle training also includes the recitation or utterance of specific mantras. Mantras can bring both subtle and spiritual results depending on the level of mantra or type, but in this book only the subtle realm is discussed. The third type of armor is spiritual, and that type of armor begins to shine when we employ specific mantras, which are sometimes defined as "sounds meant to liberate the mind from material encumbrance."

Wearing and maintaining the three types of armor well ensures a far more enjoyable and productive function of a martial artist while not denying the external approach—it merely complements it. We live in a physical and tangible world, and we need all the numbers and details that enhance a warrior's physical performance. However, that should not happen at the cost of one's quality of life, health, and happiness.

Chapter I

Ayurvedic Background

We Are Little Universes in a Grand Universe

Ayurveda, the science of life, describes five main energies, or forces, as constitutional factors of all animate and inanimate objects within the universe and, therefore, also our own bodies. These are, from most subtle to most gross, ether, air, fire, water, and earth. These building blocks form the functional energies within our own bodies, of which there are three in number: vata, pitta, and kapha. Many Ayurvedic books quote verses from *Ashtanga Hridaya*, a scripture that lists qualities and actions of the three main energies. (1.11–12)

Vata, the root of all three, consists primarily of air and secondarily of ether, which contains it. Its attributes are dryness, lightness, coldness, mobility, and roughness. Vata is the energy of movement. Vata's actions in the physical realm include maintaining homeostasis (balance), sustained exertion (effort), breathing, movement in general, and the workings of the nervous system (e.g., neural responses), and coordination of how various senses work (feet, hands, eyes, etc.). The subtle aspect, known in Sanskrit as Prana, provides us with enthusiasm, will to live, adaptability to situations, creativity, and general growth of body and mind.

Pitta consists mainly of fire and secondarily of water. Pitta's qualities are oiliness, hotness, lightness, sour smell, mobility, liquidity, and sharpness. Pitta is the energy of transformation. Its actions in the bodily realm include digestion and production of heat for all levels of combustion. On the mental platform (Tejas), pitta governs perception, understanding (intelligence), desire to learn, the quality of courage, valor, and self-discipline.

Kapha consists primarily of water and secondarily of earth. Its characteristics are wetness, coldness, heaviness, dullness, softness, steadiness, and stickiness. Kapha is the energy of cohesion. Its bodily actions are identified as giving stability, lubricating and binding together joints, and giving physical endurance for sustained work. Kapha's mental field of action (known as Ojas) is the giving of mental strength, good memory, contentment, fortitude, patience, feelings of peace, emotional and psychological stability, and strengthening of the immune system.

Three Energies in the External World

It is important to be able to observe the energies of the doshas—vata, pitta, and kapha—not only in ourselves but also in the external world. Why? Because the external world affects our world, and if we learn to discern the flow of energy in the external world, we will be able to aptly adjust our own systems to act with ease, efficiency, and joy.

The vata energy in nature can be likened to the leaves, which alter their colors and then fall from the trees. It can also be observed in the blooming of flowers and then their withering. You can also imagine trees swaying in the breeze. A gusty wind sweeps through our environment with the cold and mobile qualities of vata. When you see animals in nature, it is often because they are displaying their vata-like tendencies. This fast-paced tendency is seen in sparrows chirping and flittering about, squirrels jumping in and out of trees, rabbits quickly hopping away, and deer darting into the forest.

Pitta energy can be likened to a caterpillar emerging from a cocoon as a butterfly or a bee pollinating a flower. Think of the fruits, vegetables, and herbs that grow in your or your neighbor's garden. They grow from something very tiny into something edible. This is a natural process that requires sunshine and some moisture. Both of these elements compose pitta in the natural world. Also, pitta is hot like the rays of the sun or the sand on a beach. Pitta is like the brilliant sun, and at night, the moon and stars display pitta in their luminosity. All radiance can be described as the light of pitta. In the world of shapes, pitta is sharp like a ridge or blades of grass. Pitta's sharpness allows it to physically penetrate objects. Birds use their beaks as a tool, and elephants use their pointy tusks as a defense tool as well.

Kapha energy can be likened to a heavy mountain. Kapha is moist like the rain, the dew drops, and the snowflakes. Kapha's solidity is perceived in stones and boulders. Trees are a grand manifestation of such kapha qualities as beauty and groundedness (especially) in their trunks and roots. Wonderful waterfalls exist because of the wet and heavy qualities of kapha. The sap from trees is also kapha since it is sweet, sticky, and thick. Further examples are fog (which symbolizes thickness and slowness) and the clouds (which are heavy, slow, cool, and moist).

Although we all contain these energies within ourselves, it is the proportions, or amounts, of every one of them that make us functionally different. The vata, pitta, and kapha energies can be perceived by the bodily and mental attributes we exhibit. These varying amounts of vata, pitta, and kapha that we acquire at birth are to be maintained in the same state of equilibrium. For the sake of explaining this concept, we will call this a "harmony" or a "physiologically and psychologically happy state." It is never the goal to make their naturally varying amounts even.[1] The goal is to determine the dominant and lesser powers that move around our body-mind system and then maintain their naturally uneven levels so that our predominant powers do not usurp total control.

The ability to maintain the optimal level of life forces in our body-mind system is directly related to our awareness of factors inside and outside our body and our acting according to laws that govern them. If we do that, our martial arts will be at a superior level. Ayurveda gives us the tools in the form of powerful knowledge to assimilate into our lifestyles.

The majority of martial arts in the West seem to be flowing against the current of natural laws described in the ancient scriptures of Ayurveda. From the wrong time to get up, to the wrong kind of breakfast to eat, to the wrong time of training, and to the wrong bedtime, the martial arts we are practicing could be unnecessarily straining our body-mind system, thus throwing us off our optimal state of functioning. This may not be very evident during the course of our practice or in the beginning years. However, decades later, such a disharmonized practice will precipitate injuries, incongruous emotional states, and an overall feeling of dissatisfaction with what you do. Martial arts, as both a form of exercise and even our livelihood, should make our whole system feel better at all levels.

---

[1] In rare instances, some body-mind systems are created with even amounts of vata, pitta, and kapha, and then such an equal state should be maintained for life.

In the subsequent sections and chapters, I will present, one by one, the factors inside the body, or the small universe, the factors outside the body, the grand universe, and how to navigate through them by using them to our combative advantage.

Three Modes of Material Nature

In addition to the forces of vata,pitta, and kapha, there are three gunas, "ropes," that affect our actions on the mental field. "Material nature consists of three modes—goodness, passion, and ignorance. When the eternal living entity comes in contact with nature, O mighty-armed Arjuna, he becomes conditioned by three modes." (Bg. 4.15)

When we talk about the physical body, we talk about the doshas, and when we talk about the mind, the gunas are given primary importance. The gunas are subtle. They operate at certain times of the day, just like the doshas, and they exert a powerful influence on our minds. The mode of goodness (sattva) functions in the morning between 1 a.m. and 8 a.m., and it is the principle of intelligence. It is harmony and virtue, it has an inward and upward movement as related to our life force, and it accelerates the development of the spirit, which brings lasting enjoyment. The mode of passion (rajas) works in the late morning and into the afternoon, roughly between 9 a.m. and 4 p.m., and it is the principle of energy exemplified by activity and turbulence. It has outward orientation, causes selfishly directed activities, and brings destruction. The third mode, the mode of ignorance (tamas), operates in the evening hours of 5 p.m. until midnight and exemplifies the principle of materiality. It increases the qualities of dullness, darkness, and inertia. It has downward movement that causes disintegration, delusion, and decay.

In chapter II, "Your Individual Body Type and Mental Constitution," you will discover what your mental disposition is and which modes you are more likely to respond to. It is imperative to understand the importance of the modes, as they propel our minds into certain modes of thinking, feeling, and willing. As with the doshas and our preferred mode of appearance and action, we have our preferred ways of thinking, feeling, and willing, which, unsurprisingly, determine our subsequent actions. Like attracts like, and the predominant mode of gunas that we acquired at birth will determine the easiness or reluctance with which we respond to external forces of the three gunas.

How the Three Subtle Modes Relate to Three Gross Body Types

It is important to see the characteristics of the modes in the light of the three doshic body types because the three modes manifest different qualities in each of them. For example, goodness manifests in vata qualities such as lightness, clarity, and creativity. In pitta individuals, goodness will show in the acquirement of knowledge and understanding of concepts. In kapha persons, goodness will appear as love, compassion, and forgiveness. Passion manifests in vata individuals as hyperactivity, fear, anxiety, and ungroundedness. In pitta individuals, it will be expressed as competitiveness, aggressiveness, and desire for power and recognition. In kapha persons, it will manifest as attachment, greed, and possessiveness. Last, the mode of ignorance will display itself in vata individuals as confusion, indecisiveness, and sadness. Pitta persons will express anger, hatred, and enviousness. Kapha individuals can display a very high level of confusion, depression, and even unconsciousness.

Just as we carry a dominance of one or two body types, we will also display a tendency to show certain traits of goodness, passion, and ignorance. My spiritual master gave me a practical example as follows: An individual in the mode of goodness will think, Let me become something first and then do something so that I can obtain something (although at that point, the "getting of something" is less important and happens naturally). A person in the mode of passion will think, Let me do something so I can obtain something, and then I can become something. We can determine if we are in the mode of ignorance if we think, Let me get something so I can do something important, and then I can become something.

External Energy Flow

The flow of energies outside the body can roughly be broken down into six four-hour periods, which add up to a full day. Vata (air, ether) is dominant from 2 a.m. to 6 a.m. Kapha (earth, water) rules from 6 a.m. to 10 a.m. Pitta (fire, water) controls from 10 a.m. to 2 p.m. Vata predominates again from 2 p.m. to 6 p.m. Kapha, from 6 p.m. to 10 p.m. Pitta, from 10 p.m. to 2 a.m. Aligning our actions/activities with those times puts us in a better position to maintain harmony and life force. For example, if by constitution you are a pitta individual, ruled by fire and water, then doing an intense workout between noon and 1 p.m. may unnecessarily increase the fire element in your body and cause too much water loss. On the other hand, a workout performed in the earlier or later hours of the day, which are ruled by other elements, may prove to offer a much more pleasant experience for the whole body-mind system. It may actually balance your energetic components more for the rest of the day. We will offer more details on that in the specific chapter on training according to your constitution.

Like Activity Increases Like Energies

Your dominant energy in the body normally gravitates toward increasing itself. That is only natural, because that is the energy field familiar to your being, to your personality. For example, if you tend to be competitive in life in general and exhibit a well-developed musculature even without much work at the gym, you will naturally want to engage in various types of sports, physical activities, and competitive events of that type, as well as listen to loud and even more stimulating music. In other words, to have a sitting job that's very steady and to abhor sports feels to run against your spirit. On the other side of the spectrum, picture someone whose demeanor is rather mellow, not competitive when it comes to achieving things in life, who enjoys a milder kind of music, and who has a rather peaceful and steady job. Such a person would certainly appreciate sports like running, yoga, and tai chi but nothing like football, karate, or mixed-martial arts.

As you become aware of the three gunas working within your mind and yet outside of you, you begin to appreciate the dichotomy between yourself and the transient waves of material nature. You begin to have true observation. You will know that you are not the thoughts in your mind and that only some feelings and thoughts come directly from the spirit, from the core of your being, and the rest are stimulated by the external world and the previous baggage of desires brought about into this existence. Then you will know how to respond to such promptings and hence how to stay in harmony with your energies so that the dominant ones do not snatch the reins of your life, causing disturbance.

The Principle of Guided Acceleration

Once a warrior knows his/her dominant and subservient natures and is aware of how the external flow of energy affects them, they will adjust their daily regimen—workouts, meal times, and bedtimes included—to avoid falling out of their harmonic orbit of power. Not only that, they will choose precisely those activities that are conductive to their staying on the path of harmony. What does that mean?

It certainly does not mean that a person of fiery character should avoid competition, heated debates, and entrepreneurship altogether. These are their strengths, so why should they be neglected? Why shouldn't you fire your left hook kick if that's the best leg kick you've got? But to prevent exhaustion and to prevent your opponent from reading you easily, you don't want to be firing your best weapon every time or too often. Staying on the path of harmony means that a warrior should carefully choose the time of day to perform at their best as well as daily nurture the subservient energies that will support the dominant energies they live by. Daily nurturing the subservient energies will allow them to decelerate properly when they are about to take a turn on the road of life while the dominant energies recover.

The dominant energies will be highly effective if used sparingly according to time and circumstances of life, not most of the time. A practical example is that of a race car driver that drives around the town. The power of the car is sufficient to win a race, but when one is driving around the town to run errands, full throttle is not necessary. Actually, using the car's near maximum power while trying to obey traffic rules would prove counterproductive and destructive. The above example assumes the normal use of a vehicle is a normal "go to work, come back" type of usage, not "living on a race track." We must enable ourselves to willfully turn off and on the dominant energies of vata, pitta, or kapha so that they do not increase without control and wreak havoc. The harmonious cooperation of the threefold energies (dominant and subservient) is true strength, and their efficient manipulation lies at the heart of this manual.

We Are Not the Energies but the Energetic

The different energetic factors of vata, pitta, and kapha are the controlled, and we are sitting inside the vehicle of our body channeling the energies with our thoughts, actions, and words.[2] A suitable example is given of the

---

[2] In the science of bhakti yoga, though, the spirit contained in the physical body is understood to be the conscious energy of the Supreme Energetic Controller. In that sense, we are the energies of the Supreme Energetic. For the purpose of keeping this book at a certain platform, I chose not to digress into other explanations of the energy phenomena.

body as a chariot. The body is composed of the five great elements (earth, water, fire, air, and ether), which give rise to vata, pitta, and kapha. The senses—such as the eyes for seeing, nose for smelling, and ears for hearing—are the horses. The mind is the reins. The intelligence is the driver. The intelligence makes decisions based on our desires, and the mind brings ideas. Mind and intelligence are looked at in terms of the three modes of material nature.

Chapter II

Your Individual Body Type and Mental Constitution

We will begin by explaining the body-type paradigm. A body type denotes a particular structure (bones, muscles, etc.) and particular metabolic functioning (e.g., rate of digestion, heartbeat, etc.). Knowing your body type is just like knowing that driving a diesel will require a different fuel than driving a Honda. The modern fitness science recognizes body typings that are based mainly on the works of Dr. William H. Sheldon, who introduced the theory of somatotypes in the 1940s in *The Varieties of Human Physique*. In *The Varieties of Temperament*, Dr. Sheldon also presented three personality types. In the former, we can find descriptions of the three main body types: ectomorph (vata), mesomorph (pitta), and endomorph (kapha).

Sheldon's presentation of body types has become essential to much of the literature on exercise and bodybuilding, but the idea of body types and their corresponding psychological types did not originate with Sheldon. For example, Plato's *The Republic* and Ayurveda describe similar ideas and principles. Dr. Sheldon mentions himself that Hippocrates designated two fundamental body types. (10) Numerous French, German, Italian, and English researchers have conducted studies and postulated theories about body types. We can mention names such as Halle, Rostan, di Giovanni, Viola, and Kretschmer.

In Dr. Sheldon's work, different bodies' particular food needs according to body type are mentioned, but no conclusive recommendations are made, (248–49) and that's where the science of Ayurveda comes in with its specific nutritional recommendations. That will be given in the third chapter.

What follows is a standard but detailed questionnaire based on Ayurvedic sources I have studied. Every smart athlete determines his/her body type and trains/lives accordingly. It is good to use this questionnaire as a guide to finding your physical type and mental constitution. The first 36 questions pertain to our physical (or outer) layer, and the remaining 30 questions pertain to our mental (or inner) layer. The outer layer is best described in terms of the three doshas (vata, pitta, and kapha), and the inner layer is best described in terms of three modes of nature (sattva, rajas, and tamas).[3] The mental constitution takes precedence over the physical.

Body Type

1. What is your body's frame?

Vata (V)—	Pitta (P)—	Kapha (K)—
Unusually short or tall, thin, slim, poorly developed physique, although muscles may be very visible along with protruding veins	Medium, moderately developed physique with many visible muscles (good definition) such as the arms and stomach	Large, stout, stocky, short, well-developed physique, but muscles and veins are not visible except for the calves, chest, and forearms

---

[3] The mental tendencies and, therefore, one's mental constitution can still be described in terms of the three doshas because the doshas ultimately consist of three modes of nature in their subtle dimension. It is said that vata at the level of the mind is 75 percent mode of passion (rajas), 20 percent mode of goodness (sattva), 5 percent mode of ignorance (tamas). Similarly, it is said that pitta it is at least 50 percent mode of goodness, 45 percent passion and 5 percent ignorance. Kapha is approximately 75 percent mode of ignorance, 20 percent mode of goodness, and 5 percent passion. (Lad, 105–6)

2. If you don't exercise and eat your usual food, what weight does your body tend toward?

Vata (V)—	Pitta (P)—	Kapha (K)—
Low, with prominent veins and bones	Medium, with good musculature	Heavy, tends toward obesity

Note: Vata people can be overweight as well, but their weight will vary, and they cannot maintain the once-gained weight for very long. On the other hand, it is hard for kapha warriors to keep their weight off, as they easily store water and fat. Pitta warriors, even though of voracious appetites, usually stay at the same weight, although they can end up obese by eating greasy food and red meat.

3. What is your complexion?

Vata (V)—	Pitta (P)—	Kapha (K)—
Dull, brown, darker	Reddish, flushed, glowing	Whitish, pale

Note: We also have to consider racial differentiations. For example, African-American warriors will have a dark complexion more or less, but that does not mean that they will necessarily be vata types. Similarly, Europeans will tend to be reddish or whitish, but they may not all be pittas or kaphas.

4. How is your skin?

Vata (V)—	Pitta (P)—	Kapha (K)—
Thin, cold, rough, dry, cracked	Warm, moist, covered with moles	Thick, whitish, cold, moist, soft

Note: Skin texture is more of a determining factor than complexion is. For example, vatas will constantly have dry skin with fissures. Pitta warriors will easily burn their skin when exposed to the sun and oftentimes get rashes, sores, etc. Kaphas will always have a kind of oily, damp skin because they store more subcutaneous fat.

5. How is your hair?

Vata (V)—	Pitta (P)—	Kapha (K)—
Thin, brittle, dry, a little curly, brown	Straight, oily, early gray or bald	Thick, oily, very wavy

Note: Considering the racial characteristics, you should look more for texture and quality of hair rather than strictly the color. Vata types might often have dandruff. Pittas may often have ruddy hair and a head sensitive to sun exposure. Kapha types will usually have prominent body hair.

6. What size and shape is your head?

Vata (V)—	Pitta (P)—	Kapha (K)—
Small, elongated, thin	Medium, angular	Large, square, round

Note: How you typically move your head may be more significant in determining your type than its size and shape. Vata head movements are more erratic, usually more frequent. Vatas tend toward either excessive cervical mobility or rigidity, the two extremes. Kaphas have the least amount of cervical movement.

7. How is your face?

Vata (V)—	Pitta (P)—	Kapha (K)—
Thin, long, dull, wrinkled	Medium, sharp contours	Large, round, pale

8. How is your neck?

Vata (V)—	Pitta (P)—	Kapha (K)—
Thin, long	Medium	Stocky, thick

9. How are your eyebrows?

Vata (V)—	Pitta (P)—	Kapha (K)—
Small, thin	Medium, fine	Thick, bushy

10. How are your eye lashes?

Vata (V)—	Pitta (P)—	Kapha (K)—
Small, dry	Small, thin	Large, oily, thick

11. How are your eyes?

Vata (V)—	Pitta (P)—	Kapha (K)—
Small, active, black, brown	Medium, piercing, bright, green, red	Wide, blue, calm, attractive

Note: The eyes are an essential indicator of your type. For example, vatas' eyes have a tendency to dry out quickly and hence the tendency to constantly blink. It is a challenge for them to fix their eyes on any particular point for a longer time. Pittas are sensitive to light and often need prescription glasses and/or sunglasses. Kaphas often discharge mucus through the eyes and are more likely to release tears.

12. How is your nose?

Vata (V)—	Pitta (P)—	Kapha (K)—
Uneven, long, thin	Sharp, medium, pink	Thick, round, oily, wide nostrils

13. How are your lips?

Vata (V)—	Pitta (P)—	Kapha (K)—
Small, thin, dry, cracked	Medium, soft, red	Large, thick, smooth

14. How are your teeth and gums?

Vata (V)—	Pitta (P)—	Kapha (K)—
Thin, small, crooked	Soft, medium, bleed easily	Thick, soft, large

Note: Here, the most distinguishing factor is the color and general form of the teeth and gums. Everything else is largely influenced by our dental hygiene. For example, vata types will commonly have spaces between the teeth, whereas kaphas will feature white and large teeth.

15. How are your shoulders?

Vata (V)—	Pitta (P)—	Kapha (K)—
Small, hunched, flat	Medium	Broad, firm

16. How is your chest?

Vata (V)—	Pitta (P)—	Kapha (K)—
Flat, sunken, narrow	Medium	Expanded, broad, overly developed

17. How is your stomach?

Vata (V)—	Pitta (P)—	Kapha (K)—
Thin, sunken, visible abdominal muscles	Medium, visible abdominal muscles	Potbellied, abdominal muscles usually not visible

18. How are your arms?

Vata (V)—	Pitta (P)—	Kapha (K)—
Thin, short or long	Medium	Large, thick, round

19. How are your hands?

Vata (V)—	Pitta (P)—	Kapha (K)—
Small, thin, cold, unsteady	Medium, warm, pinkish	Large, oily, cool, firm

Note: Vatas' hands feature veins and clearly visible large knuckles. Pitta types have warm hands even when it is cold outside. Kaphas tend to have square hands without several lines.

20. How are your thighs?

Vata (V)—	Pitta (P)—	Kapha (K)—
Thin	Medium	Round, plump, developed

21. How are your hips?

Vata (V)—	Pitta (P)—	Kapha (K)—
Slender, thin	Medium	Heavy, large

22. How are your legs, in general?

Vata (V)—	Pitta (P)—	Kapha (K)—
Excessively long or short with prominent knees	Medium	Large, stocky

23. How are your calves?

Vata (V)—	Pitta (P)—	Kapha (K)—
Small, hard	Soft, loose	Firm, shaped

24. How are your feet?

Vata (V)—	Pitta (P)—	Kapha (K)—
Small (but could be long), thin, dry, unsteady	Medium, soft, pink	Large, firm, hard

Note: The dry nature of vatas will often show through the dryness of their feet, whereas pittas will have good circulation even there. Kaphas' feet are thick at the bottom.

25. How are your joints?

Vata (V)—	Pitta (P)—	Kapha (K)—
Cracking, thin, cold	Medium, soft,	Large, well-developed

Note: Vatas are characterized by prominent joints. Kapha types have significantly larger joints, but they still may be covered by excess tissue. Pittas fall in the middle, and the softness of their joints is due to excessive oils in the body.

26. How are your nails?

Vata (V)—	Pitta (P)—	Kapha (K)—
Small, dry, brittle, darker	Medium, sharp, flexible, pinkish	Large, thick, smooth, white, oily

Note: As you may know, the nails show how well we absorb our nutrients (especially minerals). Usually, vatas have the hardest time with absorption. Also, after an intense disease, the condition of our nails worsens.

27. How are your waste materials?

Vata (V)—	Pitta (P)—	Kapha (K)—
Scanty	Abundant	Moderate

Note: Vata types will normally have colorless urine and tend toward constipation, whereas pittas will have yellowish or reddish urine and tend toward diarrhea (both with a burning sensation). Kaphas will often have mucus in their metabolic wastes. As far as sweating is concerned, the vatas and kaphas will have almost no odor and scanty sweat (especially vatas), whereas pittas will have a strong body odor in profuse quantity.

28. What is your appetite like?

Vata (V)—	Pitta (P)—	Kapha (K)—
Variable, little	Strong, sharp	Slow but steady

Note: Appetite is one of the best indicators of your individual constitution. Vatas experience the extremes— that is, either no desire to eat or extreme hunger pangs— whereas kaphas are very consistent with their appetite, and they even become attached to food. Pittas tend to be voracious eaters and consume huge amounts of food without gaining weight. While hungry, vatas are induced to become fearful and feel dizzy, and pittas are induced to become angry.

29. What food do you prefer?

Vata (V)—	Pitta (P)—	Kapha (K)—
Sweet, sour, salty with oils and spices	Sweet, bitter, astringent, raw, without oil or spices	Bitter, pungent, astringent, with spices but less

Note: It is interesting to note that the above taste preferences reflect your taste preferences when you are in good balance (the five types of Chi are operating at a level close to optimal). When we are off-balance, our taste preferences change and become quite opposite to what we normally like to eat.

30. How thirsty are you throughout the day?

Vata (V)—	Pitta (P)—	Kapha (K)—
It varies	Constantly thirsty	Not very thirsty

31. How is your circulation?

Vata (V)—	Pitta (P)—	Kapha (K)—
Poor, erratic	Good, warm	Slow, steady

Note: Vatas who have weaker circulation will have a tendency to heart palpitations, and their extremities will be cold along with their abdomen. Pitta types, due to their high-level circulation, will often flush up on their face. Kaphas, on the other hand, when overweight, will weaken their peripheral circulation and also exhibit cold limbs except for the abdomen.

32. How is your daily natural mode of activity?

Vata (V)—	Pitta (P)—	Kapha (K)—
Quick, hyperactive, erratic, unsteady	Medium, goal-oriented, motivated	Slow, steady

Note: Vata individuals tend to engage in some extreme activity that will quickly exhaust them, either mentally or physically. Pitta individuals are very active and focused only when there is a purpose they've decided to fulfill. Kapha individuals, on the other hand, are steady in their actions, but they then get attached to a pattern of activity, which can be very hard to change. They often are not willing to do things very differently.

33. How is your muscular strength and exertion level?

Vata (V)—	Pitta (P)—	Kapha (K)—
Low, tendency to start and stop quickly, poor strength	Medium, average endurance, but cannot tolerate heat well	Strong, tendency to start slowly, but able to continue for a long time

Note: It is worth mentioning that vatas often become great runners (especially in long-distance running) with the ability to adapt, which is a type of strength endurance, but their lifting strength is significantly less. Pittas often like to display their power, and in the realm of sports they tend to become explosive athletes, or the so-called anaerobic athletes. Their muscular endurance tends to be mediocre. Kaphas have very good muscular endurance (quite the opposite of vatas), but their cardiovascular endurance is lacking, and thus they rarely become runners or enjoy it. In the realm of sports and fitness, they may become powerlifters or engage in strongman competitions, which require very strong muscular contractions for a relatively long time (two to five minutes with almost no break).

34. What are your environmental sensitivities?

Vata (V)—	Pitta (P)—	Kapha (K)—
Dislike cold, wind and dry weather	Dislike heat, sun and fire	Dislike cold, dampness, but like sun and wind

Note: Vatas are most sensitive to the extremes of changing weather and must therefore guard themselves properly, whereas kaphas do very well outdoors without much protection. Pittas are very tolerant of cold temperatures.

35. How is your resistance to disease?

Vata (V)—	Pitta (P)—	Kapha (K)—
Poor, changeable, low immunity	Ave. immunity, but prone to infections	Very good immune system, rarely get sick

Note: While getting sick once in a while is quite normal, the frequency of catching a common cold or flu certainly shows the quality of our nutrition and lifestyle.

36. How is your pulse?

Vata (V)—	Pitta (P)—	Kapha (K)—
Rapid, irregular, weak	Bound, moderate	Deep but slow, steady

Mental Constitution

1. How is your normal mental nature?

Vata (V)—	Pitta (P)—	Kapha (K)—
Quick, active, adaptable, indecisive	Reasoning, penetrating, critical	Slow, steady

Note: It is important to realize that our mental nature does not have to reflect our physical nature, but more often than not it does. One mental nature is not smarter than the other, but it merely displays a different kind of intelligence. For example, a vata nature would be great at abstract thinking and comparing different viewpoints, whereas a pitta nature would display a probing and scientific mentality, determining goals, ascertaining values, etc. A kapha nature is consistent and of broad principles with strong sentiments, and not very detail-oriented.

2. How is your intellectual activity?

Vata (V)—	**Pitta (P)—**	**Kapha (K)—**
Fast but often incorrect response	Accurate response	Slow but exact response

3. How is your voice?

Vata (V)—	**Pitta (P)—**	**Kapha (K)—**
Low, hoarse	High pitch, sharp	Deep, pleasant

Note: Vatas tend to have monotonous voices. Pittas make good speakers and strong singers (e.g., rock singers). Kaphas tend to have very beautiful voices and make good singers.

4. How is your speech?

Vata (V)—	**Pitta (P)—**	**Kapha (K)—**
Fast, inconsistent, tend to talk a lot	Moderate, argumentative, talk with conviction	Slow, definite, talk little

5. How is your memory?

Vata (V)—	**Pitta (P)—**	**Kapha (K)—**
Poor, notice things easily but also forget easily	Sharp, notice things clearly	Slow to take notice but do not forget

6. What is your emotional temperament?

Vata (V)—	Pitta (P)—	Kapha (K)—
Fearful, nervous	Irritable, contentious	Calm, content, sentimental

Note: Vata individuals tend to be ungrounded in their approach to life, and that encourages the fear factor and sudden shifts of thought patterns and sometimes emotions. A pitta warrior will be vehement and strong in his/her display of emotions. A kapha person will be settled and, therefore, more attached to things, persons, and ideas.

7. How strong is your resolve/discipline?

Vata (V)—	Pitta (P)—	Kapha (K)—
Changeable	Intense, extreme	Mellow but consistent

8. What are your emotional strengths?

Vata (V)—	Pitta (P)—	Kapha (K)—
Flexibility, adaptability	Fearlessness, courage	Peace, contentment

9. What is the nature of your faith in something?

Vata (V)—	Pitta (P)—	Kapha (K)—
Changeable, rebellious	Determined, extreme	Loyal, conservative

Note: Vata persons tend to be unsteady in their beliefs, or they may have faith in many different things. Pitta persons can focus their faith in a strong manner, and they have an extremist tendency in them. Kapha individuals usually have an unquestionable sense of belief and are attached to the status quo.

10. How would you describe your sleep?

Vata (V)—	Pitta (P)—	Kapha (K)—
Light, tending toward insomnia	Average, may wake up but easily fall asleep again	Heavy, difficult to wake up, like to nap during the day

11. How would you describe your dreams?

Vata (V)—	Pitta (P)—	Kapha (K)—
Flying, moving, nightmares	Colorful, full of conflict, violence	Sentimental, few dreams

12. What best describes your habits?

Vata (V)—	Pitta (P)—	Kapha (K)—
Moving, traveling, dancing, drama, joking, artistic activities	Competitive sports, politics, hunting	Spending time near water, sailing, flowers, cooking

13. How would you describe your nutrition?

Vata (V)—	Pitta (P)—	Kapha (K)—
Some meat	Heavy meat	Vegetarian

Note: It is significant to note that although meat protein builds tissue faster than vegetable or milk protein do, the tissue thus built has less endurance and resiliency. In general, vata types need more tissue-building foods than other types and therefore oftentimes resort to meat. Pitta types tend to eat denser foods such as meat because of their superior digestive strength. Kapha types already tend to have strong bones, joints, and large body mass, hence they are most likely to skip heavier foods such as meats, nuts, seeds, and milk.

14. How often do you use intoxicants such as alcohol or coffee?

Vata (V)—	**Pitta (P)—**	**Kapha (K)—**
Frequently	Occasionally	Never

15. When you go about your day and interact with people and objects, how are the impressions that they leave on your mind?

Vata (V)—	**Pitta (P)—**	**Kapha (K)—**
Disturbed	Mixed	Calm and pure

Note: The processing of mental images is known as the second level of digestion. A lot of your overall health and working energy that you are able to put out is determined by how you handle the incoming stimuli. It is therefore crucial to perform the neti pot exercise and then different types of breathing to clear the mind from its accumulated luggage. A clear mind is a must for a combat athlete. The ability to maintain a clear mind during combative practice or an actual fight is yet another level of advancement.

16. How capable are you of restraining yourself overall (e.g., not yelling at someone, forgoing the sweet on the table, etc.)?

Vata (V)—	Pitta (P)—	Kapha (K)—
Not good	Good	In the middle

17. What is your work ethic?

Vata (V)—	Pitta (P)—	Kapha (K)—
I tend to be selfless	I work mainly for personal enjoyment and close family	I have lazy work standards

18. How often do you display anger?

Vata (V)—	Pitta (P)—	Kapha (K)—
Sometimes	Frequently	Almost never

19. How often do you tend to be fearful?

Vata (V)—	Pitta (P)—	Kapha (K)—
Frequently	Rarely	Sometimes

20. What is your level of pride?

Vata (V)—	Pitta (P)—	Kapha (K)—
Modest	Excessive	Moderate

21. Do you display a tendency toward depression?

Vata (V)—	Pitta (P)—	Kapha (K)—
Frequently	Never	Sometimes

22. Are you content with life in general?

Vata (V)—	Pitta (P)—	Kapha (K)—
Partly	Never	Usually

23. How easy is it for you to forgive the faults of others?

Vata (V)—	Pitta (P)—	Kapha (K)—
I forgive easily	I forgive with effort	I hold long-term grudges

24. Describe in one word your ability to concentrate.

Vata (V)—	Pitta (P)—	Kapha (K)—
Poor	Good	Moderate

25. How is your memory?

Vata (V)—	Pitta (P)—	Kapha (K)—
Poor	Moderate	Good

26. How is your willpower?

Vata (V)—	Pitta (P)—	Kapha (K)—
Variable	Strong	Weak

27. Are you peaceful?

Vata (V)—	Pitta (P)—	Kapha (K)—
Rarely	Partially	Most of the time

28. Are you creative?

Vata (V)—	Pitta (P)—	Kapha (K)—
Very much so	Somewhat	Not usually

29. How often do you like to meditate or engage in spiritually uplifting activities?

Vata (V)—	Pitta (P)—	Kapha (K)—
Occassionally	Almost daily	Almost never

30. Do you like to serve others?

Vata (V)—	Pitta (P)—	Kapha (K)—
Very much so	Sometimes	Not really

Now that you have completed the test, add up all the Vs, Ps, and Ks, and see where you stand in the physical dimension. Next, do the same with the mental constitution. It is quite common and okay to have two dominant natures that are almost equally present. You will need to account for both of them in adjusting your daily routine and training.

The training and general mode of being that is aligned with one's mental disposition will allow for substantial advancement at the level of consciousness and provide a warrior with the best experience of the process possible. Being harmonized with your mental constitution means you keep your dominant energies under control while feeding the subservient minor energies. In light of the previous chapter, we could provide the example of a battery and the electric current. The current will flow efficiently when positive and negative ends are connected. The current will not flow when either two positives or two negatives are connected. When you keep adding and adding to your already dominant tendencies, they will disable you from feeling harmony, whereas giving the dominant tendencies a break and feeding the minor tendencies will truly empower your dominant side.

Chapter III

Physical Armor

Building Blocks for Body and Mind per Body Type

Vata (V)—	Pitta (P)—	Kapha (K)—
Unusually short or tall, thin, slim, poorly developed physique, although muscles may be very visible along with protruding veins.	Medium, moderately developed physique with many visible muscles (good definition) such as arms and stomach.	Large, stout, stocky, short, well-developed physique, but muscles and veins are not visible except for calves, chest, and forearms.

Food and Mental Equilibrium

The key to productive training is healthy nutrition, and healthy nutrition is unique to each body type. Body-type-specific nutrition cannot be neglected. Each and every one of us is made of a slightly different concentration of the five elements (earth, water, etc.) and, therefore, the three doshas (vata, pitta, and kapha) at gross (physical) and subtle (mind, intelligence) levels. Similarly, different species of vegetables, grains, etc. have different concentrations of the five elements. If you know how such foods affect your body type, you will have made progress in harmonious living and also training (see appendix II for the advantages of plant-based nutrition). The father of ancient medicine, Hippocrates, has noted that

> it appears to me necessary to every physician to be skilled in nature, and strive to know...what man is in relation to the articles of food and drink, and to his other occupations, and what are the effects of each of them to everyone.... Whoever does not know what effect these things produce upon a man cannot know the consequences which result from them.... How can he understand the diseases which befall a man? For, by every one of these things, a man is affected and changed this way or that, and

the whole of his life is subjected to them, whether in health, convalescence, or disease.[4]

In *Nutrition and Your Mind*, Dr. George Watson, a renowned clinical psychologist, said that "when one knows nothing of nutrition and eats merely from ignorance, habit, and learned prejudices, there is a steady decrease in physical—and often mental—performance as the years of youth go by." (65)

When it comes to eating, a warrior has three options: one great, one good, and one not so good. They are eating for optimum health, eating for performance, and eating for survival. Most of you reading this book will not eat for survival but for enhancing your optimal health or even maximizing your combative performance. But most of the diets used by the general population can be classified as "survival eating."

The Dietary Reference Intakes are based on population averages and are supposed to determine the national health average, not the individual health average. (Gastelu and Hatfield, 12) Many progressive nutritionists confirm what the ancient medical scriptures already state, namely that our bodies need whole, fresh foods for optimal functioning. This is so because whole foods simply have more life force and nutrients than the body needs.

---

[4] This is quoted in Madej, *Krishna Warrior Fitness Challenge*, 133.

When you choose to eat for performance, quite another level of eating, you must realize that such practice may not necessarily correlate with eating for achieving harmonious balance of Chi in your life. Training mostly the body with great intensity and fueling it with powerful supplements meant to accelerate certain natural processes is certainly meant to burn out the life force of your system quicker in exchange for accelerated results in terms of power, speed, and agility. Ayurvedic science does not recommend such an approach.

If you cannot give up the performance-oriented athletic lifestyle, you can still use Ayurvedic science to derive great tips and additional knowledge on how to channel, manage, and augment your unique body-type system. You will be able to relax and rejuvenate more effectively in the off-season.

Ayurveda teaches that a vata or pitta person's nutrition should ideally consist of 50 percent body-type-specific whole grains (see food charts below), 20 percent body-type-specific protein, and 20 to 30 percent body-type-specific fresh vegetables (optional 10 percent for fresh fruit). Kaphas should eat 30 to 40 percent body-type-specific whole grains, 20 percent body-type-specific protein, and 40 to 50 percent fresh vegetables (with an optional 10 percent for fresh or dried fruit). (Lad, 82, 96)

Nutrition by Body Type and Mental Constitution

In light of the previous chapter, we can see how the physical and mental constitution can determine our nutrition. Your physical type and how it is attuned to environmental changes will affect how you metabolize, or digest, certain foods. Therefore, no single nutritional plan is good for everyone. If you have become sick and tired of counting calories, points, and grams and watching out for the glycemic index of foods, then this is a simple and comprehensive plan for you. All you need to know is your body type and mental constitution. Next, go shopping for locally grown foods, organic foods, and home-grown foods that match the chart.

Vata-Balancing Foods

Vata types, as mentioned above, will do well on a quality nutritional regimen of even up to 50 percent whole grains, leaving about 30 percent for protein foods and only 20 percent for fresh vegetables and fruit.

Food Group	Consume	Avoid
Fruit	Mostly sweet Fruits: Apples (cooked), Applesauce, Avocados, Bananas, Berries, Coconuts, Grapes, Grapefruit, Lemons, Mangos, Melons, Oranges, Papaya, Peaches, Pineapples, Plums, Raisins, Strawberries	Dried Fruits
Vegetables	Cooked vegetables: Asparagus, Carrots, Green beans, Leeks, Okra, Olives (black), Parsnip, Peas, Pumpkins, Squash (summer and winter), Sweet potatoes, Watercress, Zucchini	Frozen, Raw or Dried Vegetables
Grains	Durham flour, Essene bread, Oats (cooked), Pancakes, Quinoa, Rice (all types), Sprouted wheat, Wheat	Barley, Bread (yeasted), Buckwheat, Cereals (dried and puffed), Corn, Crackers, Granola, Muesli, Rye
Legumes	Mung beans	All other beans

Food Group	Consume	Avoid
Dairy	Most dairy products that are either raw or cold-temperature pasteurized: Butter, Cheese (soft), Clarified butter (ghee), Cottage cheese, Cow's milk, Goat's milk	Powdered milk, Yogurt (plain and frozen)
Animal foods	Chicken, Duck, Eggs, Fish (freshwater or sea), Salmon, Sardines, Seafood, Shrimp	Beef, Lamb, Pork, Venison, Turkey (white)
Condiments	Kelp, Ketchup, Lemons, Lime pickles, Mayonnaise, Mustard, Pickles, Salt, Scallions, Seaweed, Tamari, Vinegar (apple cider)	Chocolate, Horseradish
Nuts	All types	
Seeds	Chia, Flax, Pumpkin, Sesame, Sunflower, Tahini	Popcorn
Oils	Most oils, especially Sesame	
Beverages	Almond milk, Aloe vera juice, Apple cider, Carrot juice, Hot Chai, Lemonade, Rice milk	Apple juice, Black tea, Caffeinated drinks, Carbonated drinks, Chocolate milk,

Food Group	Consume	Avoid
Beverages (continued)	Sour juices (freshly made)	Coffee, Cranberry juice, Dairy drinks (cold), Iced tea, Mixed vegetable juice (V8), Pomegranate juice, Soy milk
Sweeteners	Fructose, Fruit juice concentrates, Raw honey, Molasses, Rice syrup, Sucanat, Turbinado sugar	White sugar
Supplements	Amino acids, Bee pollen, Blue-green algae, Copper, Iron, Magnesium, Spirulina, Vitamins A, Vitamin B complex, Vitamin C, Vitamin D, Vitamin E, Zinc	Barley green, Brewer's yeast
Ayurvedic Supplements	Ashwagandha, Triphala, Jatamamsi, Shilajit, Kapikacchu, Kava Kava, Myrrh	

Pitta-Balancing Foods

As mentioned earlier, pittas will do well on a quality nutritional regimen of even up to 50 percent whole grains, leaving about 20 percent for protein foods and 30 percent for fresh vegetables and fruit.

Food Group	Consume	Avoid
Fruit	Apples, Applesauce, Avocados, Berries, Coconuts, Grapes (red, purple), Mangos, Melons, Oranges, Peaches, Pineapples, Plums, Raisins, Watermelons	Sour Fruits
Vegetables	Sweet and bitter vegetables: Artichokes, Asparagus, Bitter melon, Broccoli, Brussels sprouts, Cabbages, Carrots (cooked), Cauliflower, Celery, Cucumbers, Leafy greens, Lettuce, Mushrooms, Okra, Olives (black), Parsley	Pungent vegetables: Beets (raw), Chilies (green), Garlic, Horseradish,

Food Group	Consume	Avoid
Vegetables (continued)	Peas, Potatoes, Sweet peppers, Sweet potatoes, Squash, Wheatgrass sprouts, Zucchini	Mustard greens, Olives (green), Onions (raw), Tomatoes, Spinach (raw)
Grains	Amaranth, Barley, Cereal (dry), Couscous, Crackers, Durham flour, Essene bread, Granola, Oat bran, Oats (cooked), Pancakes, Pasta, Rice (white), Rice cakes, Spelt, Tapioca, Wild rice, Wheat, Wheat bran	Bread (yeasted), Buckwheat, Corn, Millet, Oats (dry), Quinoa, Rice (brown), Rye
Legumes	Most beans	Miso, Soy sauce, Soy sausage
Dairy	Butter (unsalted), Cheese (soft and unsalted), Clarified butter (ghee), Cottage cheese, Cow's milk (raw), Goat's milk, Ice cream	Butter (salted), Buttermilk, Cheese (hard, aged), Sour cream, Yogurt (plain or frozen)
Animal foods	Chicken (white), Egg whites, Fish (freshwater), Turkey (white), Venison	All others

Food Group	Consume	Avoid
Condiments	Coriander, Sprouts	Chili pepper, Chocolate, Horseradish, Ketchup, Lemon, Lime pickle, Mayonnaise, Mustard, Salt, Scallions, Seaweed, Soy sauce, Vinegar
Nuts	Almonds soaked in purified water, Coconut	Almonds with skin, Cashews, Filberts, Macadamia nuts, Peanuts, Walnuts
Seeds	Flax, Sunflower	Chia, Tahini, Sesame
Oils	Flaxseed, Clarified butter (ghee), Olive, Soy, Sunflower, Walnut	Almond, Corn, Safflower, Sesame
Beverages	Almond milk, Aloe vera juice, Apple juice, Black tea, Carob, Dairy drinks (cool), Grain "coffee," Grape juice, Mango juice,	Apple cider, Caffeinated drinks, Carbonated drinks, Carrot juice, Chocolate milk, Coffee, Cranberry juice, Grapefruit juice, Iced tea, Lemonade, Tomato juice,

Food Group	Consume	Avoid
Beverages (continued)	Mixed vegetable juice, Peach nectar	Sour juices (pineapple), V8 juice
Sweeteners	Barley malt, Fructose, Fruit juice concentrates, Maple syrup, Rice syrup, Sucanat, Turbinado sugar	Honey, Molasses, White sugar
Supplements **Ayurvedic Supplements**	Aloe vera juice, Barley green, Blue-green algae, Brewer's yeast, Calcium, Magnesium, Spirulina, Vitamin D, Vitamin E, Zinc Amalaki, Aloe gel, Arjuna, Bala, Brahmi, Gotu kola, Shatavari	Amino acids, Copper, Iron, Vitamin A, Vitamin B complex, Vitamin C

Kapha-Balancing Foods

Kaphas will thrive on a high-quality nutritional regimen of as much as 50 percent fresh vegetables and fruit, 30 percent whole grains, and 20 percent protein foods.

Food Group	Consume	Avoid
Fruit	Apples, Applesauce, Apricots, Berries, Cherries, Cranberries, Pears, Persimmons, Pomegranates, Prunes, Raisins	Avocados, Bananas, Coconuts, Dates, Grapefruit, Kiwi, Melons, Oranges, Papayas, Pineapples, Plums, Rhubarb, Watermelons
Vegetables	Pungent and bitter vegetables: Artichokes, Asparagus, Beets, Broccoli, Cabbage, Carrots, Cauliflower, Celery, Chilis (green), Eggplant, Garlic, Green beans, Horseradish	Sweet and juicy vegetables: Cucumbers, Olives, Pumpkin, Squash (winter), Sweet potatoes, Tomatoes (raw), Zucchini

Food Group	Consume	Avoid
Vegetables (continued)	Kale, Leafy greens, Leeks, Lettuce, Mushrooms, Okra, Onions, Parsley, Potatoes (white), Spinach, Sprouts, Tomatoes (cooked), Turnips, Watercress, Wheatgrass, Sprouts	
Grains	Barley, Buckwheat, Cereal (dry, puffed), Couscous, Crackers, Essene bread, Granola, Millet, Muesli, Oat bran, Oats (dry), Polenta, Rye, Tapioca, Wheat bran	Bread (yeasted), Oats (cooked), Pancakes, Rice, Wheat
Legumes	Adzuki beans, Black beans, Chickpeas, Lentils (red, brown), Lima beans, Navy beans, Peas (dried), Soy milk, Split peas, Tempeh, White beans	Kidney beans, Miso, Soybeans, Soy cheese, Soy flour, Soy powder, Soy sauce, Tofu (cold)
Dairy	Cottage cheese from skimmed goat's milk, Goat's milk (skim), Yogurt (diluted)	Butter, Cheese, Cow's milk, Ice cream, Sour cream, Yogurt (plain or frozen)

Food Group	Consume	Avoid
Animal foods	Chicken (white), Duck, Eggs, Fish (freshwater), Rabbit, Shrimp, Turkey (white), Venison	Beef, Buffalo, Chicken (dark), Duck, Fish (saltwater), Lamb, Pork, Sardines, Turkey (dark)
Condiments	Black pepper, Chili pepper, Horseradish, Mustard, Scallions, Sprouts	Chocolate, Kelp, Lime pickle, Mayonnaise, Pickles, Salt, Soy sauce, Tamari, Vinegar
Nuts		All
Seeds	Chia, Popcorn (no salt or butter)	Sesame, Tahini
Oils	Almond, Clarified butter (ghee), Corn, Sesame, Sunflower	Coconut, Olive, Primrose, Safflower, Sesame, Soy, Walnut
Beverages	Aloe vera juice, Apple cider, Black tea, Carob, Carrot juice, Cherry juice, Cranberry juice, Grape juice, Mango juice, Peach nectar, Pomegranate juice, Prune juice, Soy milk (hot and spiced)	Almond milk, Caffeinated drinks, Carbonated drinks, Chocolate milk, Coffee, Dairy drinks (cold), Grapefruit juice, Iced tea,

Food Group	Consume	Avoid
Beverages (continued)		Icy cold drinks, Orange juice, Rice milk, Soy milk (cold), Tomato juice, V8 Juice
Sweeteners	Fruit juice concentrates, Honey (raw and unprocessed)	Fructose, Maple syrup, Molasses, Rice syrup, Turbinado sugar, White sugar
Supplements	Aloe vera juice, Amino acids, Barley green, Blue-green algae, Brewer's yeast, Copper, Calcium, Iron, Magnesium, Vitamin A, Vitamin B, Vitamin C, Vitamin D, Vitamin E, Zinc	Potassium
Ayurvedic Supplements	Aloe gel, Arjuna, Ashwagandha, Guggul, Kava kava, Shankhapushpi, Shilajit	

Three Foods for Three Armors

Now that you have gone shopping and gotten many of the body-type-specific foods, it is time to differentiate among the foods our system requires for achievement of its ultimate function. Gross foods in the form of vegetables, protein, and fats, as well as physical exercise (martial arts or asana), directly charge the physical armor while indirectly supporting/affecting the mind and spirit. The subtle body in the form of mind and intelligence, or the subtle armor, is best charged by breathing exercises (pranayama), less directly charged by meditation, and minutely charged by gross food.[5] The spiritual armor, which is the self, or "I," is rejuvenated primarily by meditation, secondarily by pranayama, and very minutely by gross food. As you may recall from the introduction, the Internal Training Approach (ITA) that I present in *Smart Chi* obeys this principle.

It has often been my experience that individuals who are under stress tend to indulge in various foods at night to sort of feel good at the end of the day. That throws them off of their nutritional regimen as well as their pathway to health and fitness. They usually do not lose the intended weight or gain the sufficient muscle or achieve the desired muscle definition. What is happening

---

[5] The herbs and herbal preparations mentioned mainly as Ayurvedic supplements have a greater effect on the brain and mind than on the rest of the physical body.

is the stressed and overstimulated mind is taking over their taste buds and stomach and then dictating what and how much to eat. By eating in this fashion, we may balance the mind a little at the moment, but the body will be off-balance and the mind not so happy later on. The process will be repeated every time we are exposed to stress and bad feelings.

If the mind does not know how to deal with stress or how to effectively neutralize the accumulated stress, the body will never follow an optimal and healthy nutritional lifestyle. The simple solution is to allow ourselves a short 15-minute yoga session with some breathing at the end before eating dinner. You will notice the difference in mind control and your eating manner. Sitting down at a table like this, you will eat according to your actual physical needs. Breathe for the mind and eat for the body. This brings us to the next chapter.

How to Eat If You Are a Mixed Type

One may intelligently ask, "If I am a combination of two types, which do I need to eat for?" The answer is that if you are predominantly one type, your nutrition should reflect that, but if you are more in between, then the nutrition should be switched up. How?

Ayurveda teaches a seasonal approach to nutrition, and seasons reflect a certain state of energies in the universe. Summer is more like pitta, fall is more like vata, spring is more like kapha/pitta, and winter is more like vata/kapha. Let's say you are a vata-pitta. It follows then that for a vata-pitta person, in order to keep those dominant energies in balance, during the vata season one would consume more vata-pacifying foods, and during the pitta season one would use more of the pitta-pacifying foods.

Of course, environmental/climatic factors are not the only factors affecting our systems. A warrior striving for optimal health and performance must consider, in addition to the already discussed physiological and nutritional factors, his/her emotional factors. That is more directly augmented by the practice of breathing techniques (pranayama) and the chanting of mantras (mantra-yoga) and will be discussed in the chapters to follow.

Chapter IV

Subtle Armor

Rediscovering the Secret Knowledge of Ancient Masters

It is said that a great martial artist should know himself first. It is essential for any athlete, especially a combat athlete, and for any human being, for that matter, to daily monitor the level of his/her Prana. Merely asking one's trainee, "How do you feel today?" before embarking on a demanding workout is awfully vague and not of much use. A systematic questionnaire should be established where the question "How are your five Pranas flowing today?" is asked.

When we talk about Prana, or life force, we can have in mind the universal force that moves everything, like the air, seasons, planets, etc. Also, Prana can mean our own life force underlying all our activities, which can be highly enhanced by the right kind of breathing exercises.

Thus, everything that has spirit in it—like us, animals, and plants—is a little universe with its own Prana center.

Let me briefly explain here that when we breathe in air, we do not take in Prana in the literal sense of the word. The air is a raw material like coal. What occurs is that we merely take in the oxygenated air, so our own life force extracts life force from air for individual use. Through the process of breathing, our own life force rejuvenates the physical body by giving it even more life force. Place coal in the fire and you will get more heat and fire. We will discuss some powerful ways to breathe that optimize our functioning as human beings and martial artists. Now we'll talk about the five airs.

Five Types of Chi

There are five types of the same Chi—Prana—or Vayu (wind), flowing in our body-mind system according to their different powers and movement orientations. They are vividly described in some books of Ayurvedic knowledge such as the books by Dr. David Frawley (Vamadeva Shastri). One should be able to quickly assess the states of one's five Chis and be able to adjust them if needed for optimal daily functioning.

Prana Vayu.
This is our master energy. Prana means "forward" and relates to absorption. Its external aspect is located mainly

in the head and brain, and its movement oscillates among the head, throat, and chest. Its internal aspect relates to the mind and consciousness. This primary Vayu directs all the other Vayus in the body. It is responsible for having a positive attitude, taking in impressions from the outside world, receiving neural sensory impulses, receiving knowledge, processing feelings (linked to our intelligence), and, in general, collecting and energizing the external air, food, and water. As such, Prana Vayu has a mainly inward movement. When this Prana is in abundance, hardly any disease can do us harm. Enhancing this Prana is helpful in treating brain fatigue, sinus allergies, head colds, and a plethora of ailments of the nervous system.

Udana Vayu.
This is our "upward moving" or "ascending" wind. It functions mainly in the chest and throat. On the external level, Udana Vayu is in charge of speech. Internally, it governs memory, will, and effort. It also manifests as self-expression in our work and life in general. Udana Vayu also helps us manifest our life's aspirations, and when given a chance to develop to its full capacity, it can let us transcend all barriers of material nature arising from having a physical body and subtle mind. Some people possess various psychic powers, and those also exemplify a high level of Udana Vayu. This particular Prana allows for very deep abilities to discriminate and as such is linked to our intellect. Developing Udana Vayu will help protect against sore throat and a multitude of

ailments in the throat region. It greatly improves the strength and endurance of one's voice. In the karate practice, we usually end a combination with a warrior yell (Japanese: *kiai*), and Udana Vayu aids in that immensely.

Samana Vayu.
This "equalizing" or "centering" Vayu balances higher and lower body parts and their energies. Located in the small intestine, it governs digestion and assimilation. Samana Vayu dominates in the internal organs such as the stomach, liver, pancreas, and spleen, but its action covers all the internal organs in the aspect of absorption. Strong Samana Vayu means good digestion, which is an essential part of health.

Vyana Vayu.
Vyana means "diffusing" or "expanding." Its center is in the heart region, from where it channels itself to the whole body. Vyana Vayu controls both the circulatory and musculoskeletal systems in our body. As such, it internally energizes mostly the motor organs of action such as the legs and arms. What may be of particular interest for martial artists and athletes in general is that when Vyana Vayu is impaired, we will lack in coordination and movement. This form of Prana allows us to exercise and do combative training.

Apana Vayu.
This form of Prana is "moving downward," or "descending."

Its mainstay is the colon and bladder, where externally it governs elimination and urination, thus getting rid of accumulated toxins. In this way, Apana Vayu supports the other forms of Vayu. It is a descending force of deterioration that is a factor to consider whenever there is loss of strength (e.g., due to an intense workout schedule) or excessive toxins in the body (e.g., due to stress). Apana Vayu is like a plug in the body that can let the toxins out, but if it is slow, it holds the toxins in the body, contributing to disease. We must remember that our physical bodies are connected to the earth element, being composed of it, and as such we have a natural tendency to deteriorate physically just as we have a natural tendency to ascend spiritually (using the other forms of Prana). Apana Vayu internally helps us neutralize negativity from other people by being detached from it and not reacting to it.

A wise martial artist should be able to monitor and keep in balance the five Chis through individualized breathing techniques that precede and complete one's individualized yoga practices. It is important to note that although the function of the five Chis is localized, the five Chis are subtle in nature and therefore are all-pervading. They connect at all levels. Indeed, it is their goal to do that. Yet Apana Vayu (downward force of elimination) can be said to work in opposition to Udana Vayu (upward expanding force), while Vyana Vayu (outward expanding force) works in opposition to Samana Vayu (inward contracting force). Prana Vayu and Apana Vayu work more on the outside of the body whereas Samana Vayu and Vyana Vayu work within the body and the field of Prana and Apana.

The Five Vayus Related to Physical Tissues and Channels

Our bodily vehicle consists of seven tissue layers (*dhatus*): plasma (skin included), blood, muscle, fat, bone, marrow (nerve tissue included), and reproductive tissue. It is interesting to note that each of the five types of Chi has a specific effect on one of the bodily tissues. For instance, Prana Vayu enhances the marrow and nerve tissue. Udana Vayu improves the muscle tissue. Samana Vayu produces the fat tissue. Vyana Vayu optimizes the connective tissue (ligaments). Apana Vayu strengthens the bone tissue.

As far as the bodily organs are concerned, Ayurveda lists seven additional physiological systems, such as the skeletal, digestive, and nervous systems. Prana Vayu is said to function in and optimize the brain, heart, and senses (touch, smell, etc.). Udana Vayu functions in the throat, lungs, and stomach. Samana Vayu acts in the digestive organs such as the small intestine, liver, pancreas, and stomach. Vyana Vayu functions mainly in the lungs and heart, though it also functions on the periphery of the body-mind system. Apana Vayu optimizes the lower organs such as the kidneys, urinary bladder, and reproductive mechanisms. (Frawley, *Yoga and Ayurveda*, 129)

Breathing Techniques in Traditional Yoga

Controlling the breath (Sanskrit: *pranayama*) refers to injecting more life force into your system and enhancing its natural flow. Pranayama, however, is only one of the eight steps of the original Ashtanga yoga. It is certainly worthwhile to elaborate on each step a little bit for two reasons. First, every martial artist can ascend higher into the realm of perfect mind, body, and spirit, without doing which their art has little meaning. Second, much of the yoga practices in the West omit many of the more advanced and essential steps of the original Ashtanga yoga. In traditional yoga, the student goes further into levels six, seven, and eight.

Step I. *Yama* (Right Attitude).
There are five "disciplines" the yoga student practices diligently: nonviolence, truthfulness, control of sexual energy, non-stealing, and detachment (non-clinging). Following them will allow our mind and intellect to evolve and become fortified with qualities such as determination, reason,

moderation, and compassion. Such qualities will prove to be very helpful in the more advanced yoga practice.

Step II. *Niyama* (Right Action).
There are five "restraints" the yoga student practices: contentment, purity, self-study, self-discipline, and surrender to a higher power (e.g., God). We can say that many of the *yamas* and *niyamas* are very much present in traditional martial arts as well. True martial arts teachers know that if the student's manner of action is not harmonized, he/she will not have a strong foundation for achieving anything of enduring value in the arts, what to speak of life in general.

Step III. *Asana* (Physical Postures).
The third step is the practicing of physical postures, which roughly correlates with the physical training aspect of martial arts. The asanas' goal is to bring balance to the musculoskeletal system of the physical body. Therefore, they are used to increase the vital Prana and to balance the three energies of vata, pitta, and kapha. It is worth mentioning that every time your mind does not follow your breath during exercise, especially during yoga, you are minimizing the effect of that asana, which is an exercise in the process of energy harmonization. In the context of this book, we can say that if martial artists know their body type and mental constitution, they can practice the right asanas or even martial arts techniques that align more with their energy flow and type.

Step IV. *Pranayama* (Breath Control).

In the fourth stage, the yoga adept, while maintaining the above practices, places emphasis on the development and expansion of Prana. In general, one tries to deepen the breath until a peaceful condition is achieved wherein one's senses (eyes, ears, etc.), emotions, and stubborn mind are pacified just like a snake is pacified by a charmer.

Step V. *Pratyahara* (Control of the Senses).

This stage means a withdrawal from distraction, like a tortoise that withdraws its limbs. This by no means necessitates that one go to the forest and live in a cave, thus retiring from all family and social life. In this stage, one is strongly present in every situation, giving it his/her best because one is fully aware. One merely withdraws one's attention from the sensory field while the mind and intellect are present. Yoga students use mantras or visible artifacts to redirect their attention and may practice this whole program (starting with step three) in a special meditation hall. In the context of the topic of this book, such a rare state is strongly recommended in combat, when one can make clear decisions with a calm mind and therefore be most effective. One should be beyond anger, frustration, and fear when fighting one's opponent, and this is almost impossible unless one takes a comprehensive approach to one's combative practice.

Step VI. *Dharana* (Control of the Mind).
Here, the student really sharpens his/her attention on the object of yoga (the universal light, a personal form of God, the spirit in the heart or soul, etc.) so that it is one-pointed. Techniques used include focusing on ideas, specific sounds (mantras), specific objects (yantras), or the seven energy centers (chakras).

Step VII. *Dhyana* (Meditation).
Meditation is to remain focused continuously on the object of yoga. This advanced stage is a sort of trance, and one truly perceives life in a different dimension, having ascended to the natural state of awareness. The meditation can still be on the external object—such as the sky, the ocean, or a picture or statue of a deity (e.g., Buddha, Jesus, Krishna)—but the internal state is such that the object has penetrated one's consciousness and become part of one's self. Indeed, one may have visions of or revelations from the object of meditation and may no longer need the external object for meditation, especially now that it is already instilled in one's being. The student is a true master, having completely crossed over the ocean of material energy and completely identified himself/herself with the spirit.

Step VIII. *Samadhi* (Absorption).
This level indicates a total unification with the object of yoga. One may say it is the unity of the perceiver with the perceived in which direct perception takes place and

the reality of life is revealed. As such, it takes the practitioner to the underlying spiritual/divine nature of all things in ourselves and the universe.[6]

Authentic yoga teachers agree that without breath awareness, one's asana training, or martial arts techniques and forms, for that matter, have little meaning. Once you are well aware of your breathing, you are in a good position to control it and control your mind. With that, you can easily control your physical vehicle, the body, along with its senses. Many martial arts masters ascend and teach combative arts at this level of sense control, which is level five of yoga, or *pratyahara*.

Breathing Techniques for Martial Artists by Body Type

All sorts of breathing models and variations exist both in yoga and in martial arts systems. In general, the breathing technique should balance the five types of Chi and ensure their proper flow. What we will present here first is what type of breathing will be most likely to balance your individual constitution, or dosha, and also when should it be done.

---

[6] Such an enlightened human being can then choose to come out of the trance and teach others the path, or leave the physical body and transfer himself to another plane of existence.

In the morning, the mind is calmer due to the energy of goodness (sattva), and you will get the most out of your breathing and yoga practice. Pranayama should be done with fresh air, not inside a closed room, and in the morning before (for a shorter session) or after (for a longer session) yoga practice. At least crack your window open.[7] Recycled air will not do quite the same job. It is very good to clean one's nasal passages and stimulate the energy points near the nasal passages before attempting to breathe. These quick enhancement tips are given in chapter VII in "Quick Ways to Replenish Lost Chi."

In general, breathing in through the right nostril and out through the left increases fiery energy, pitta, and is thus especially beneficial for vata- and kapha-dominate types. Inhaling through the left nostril and exhaling via the right increases the energy of water and earth (kapha), which will clear the minds of pitta-dominant warriors. Alternate-nostril breathing equalizes the functioning of both energies and is recommended before morning yoga practice, but it should not be mixed with other types of breathing.

More specifically, the breathing process of pranayama consists of four phases, or parts: inhalation, inner retention (while holding air in the lungs), exhalation, and outer retention (when air is out of the lungs). Inhalation

---

[7] When it's freezing outside, you can slightly open the window and stand further away from it or open it in another room, but leave the door partially opened so the current of fresh air gets there.

increases Prana Vayu. Inner retention optimizes Samana Vayu. The point at which one approaches exhalation relates to Vyana Vayu. The first part of exhalation enhances Udana Vayu. Finally, the second part of exhalation harmonizes Apana Vayu. In terms of the doshas, inhalation increases the energy of kapha (water), inner retention increases the energy of pitta (fire), and exhalation optimizes vata (air).

The strength of one's breathing practice will be determined largely by the proportion of inhalation, exhalation, and retention. In the beginning, a one-to-two ratio is recommended. That means one should try to prolong exhalation so that it is twice as long as the time it takes to inhale. There is no focus on inner retention, or one can retain for as long as it took to inhale. In the more advanced stage, one should retain air after inhalation (inner retention) for twice as long as it took to inhale, exhale for twice as long, and retain after exhalation (outer retention) twice as long. Yet a still more advanced level is prolonging inner retention to four times the time of inhalation, exhaling for twice as long as inhalation, and holding without air (outer retention) for four times longer than inhalation. (Frawley, *Ayurveda, Nature's Medicine,* 278–79)

Every phase of breathing is essential because when one is neglected, the others will suffer. They are a family. The *Tao Te Ching* hints at what could easily describe the soft and hard breathing techniques that are delineated later in this chapter:

That which shrinks [exhalation]
  must first expand [inhalation].
That which fails [outer retention]
  must first be strong [inner retention].
That which is cast down [exhalation]
  must first be raised [inhalation].
Before receiving [inhalation of Prana]
  there must be giving [exhalation and channeling of
  Prana].
This is called perception of the nature of things.
Soft and weak overcome hard and strong
  [after each harder exhalation there must come
  inhalation, which relaxes tension in the body]. (36)

Cooling Forms of Pranayama

These should be practiced especially by pittas and, to a lesser degree, vatas. Considering the heating effect of a martial arts workout, we can also recommend them for all body types according to need, place, and circumstance.

Chandra bhedana (moon-piercing breath) entails a left-nostril inhalation (closing the right), and a short or no retention (to prevent from building up more fire). What follows is an exhalation via the right nostril. A set of a dozen or more repetitions is recommended, but it could be more depending on the individual need.

Shitali (cooling breath) involves sticking out the tongue and folding it into a tube. Then, one presses the lips around the tongue as if about to sip water. Inhalation should be deep and should generate a cooling energy in the mouth and stomach. Internal retention is maintained up to a comfortable moment, after which one exhales through both nostrils. A set of a dozen or more repetitions is good to do, but it could be more depending on one's need.

Alternate-nostril breathing is known as the most important breathing method in Ayurveda, and we will explain it in a little more detail. (Frawley, *Yoga and Ayurveda*, 249–51; Frawley, *Ayurveda, Nature's Medicine*, 283–84) It should be done after cleaning one's nasal passages with a neti pot (detailed later in this chapter) in the morning, even before one's yoga practice, or it can be done throughout the day as needed. It is the most important treatment method because it harmonizes Prana and Apana Vayus (especially in the head region), the two most important Vayus in the body.

It is important to note that the right side of the body is ruled by pitta, or fire, and it contains digestive organs (liver, pancreas), whereas the left side contains organs that nourish the whole body (e.g., the heart, stomach). The right side is dominated by the solar/heating and catabolic principle, whereas the left side is dominated by the lunar/cooling and anabolic principle. The right side stimulates the breakdown of things (sympathetic nervous system), and the left side builds and calms everything down (parasympathetic nervous system). Alternate-nostril breathing balances the energies around the main organs on both sides of the body. Thus, it is a very good method to facilitate the control of the breath and purify the various energy channels (*nadis*).

As you may or may not be aware, throughout the day, our breathing usually dominates in either one of the nostrils. When the external conditions are hot and humid, the body naturally senses it and narrows the right nostril, so the air gets inside mainly through the left passage, thus cooling the body. When the body senses that conditions outside are cold, it does the opposite to facilitate the warming process.[8] Sometimes, when you may be in doubt as to what kind of breathing method to use, by pinching one nostril and trying to breathe through the other only, you can test which nostril is more open than the other. If the left nostril is more open, that would indicate that body wants to cool down, and you may adopt a *shitali* breath to aid the body.

Begin by pinching the left nostril with the right pinky and ring finger while drawing air through the right nostril. Retain for about twice as long as it took to inhale, block the right nostril with right thumb, and exhale via the left nostril. With practice you can progress to retain

---

[8] Another example of this phenomenon is that after eating a meal, the body will switch to right-nostril breathing so that more heat is created to aid in digesting the food.

air for a longer period of time, up to the point of perspiring. Next, reverse the breathing and start by pinching the right nostril with right thumb while drawing air via the left nostril. Continue on for two to five minutes. Increase time as needed.

Heating Forms of Pranayama

Heating forms of breathing should generally be practiced by vata types and kapha types in preparation for the day of a martial arts event. They should be practiced after the alternate-nostril breathing and after one's constitutional yoga practice. When practicing breathing techniques, it is essential to maintain an erect spine (whether sitting or standing).

Kapalabhati (breath that makes the head shine) does not involve retention, but it still belongs to the heating forms of breathing. One either sits or stands in a comfortable position and performs a forceful exhalation that is slightly deeper than his/her normal breathing. The abdominal wall will momentarily and dynamically contract, after which one normally inhales. A warrior performs a set of close to a dozen exhalations. Each time, a stroke or a dynamic press to the center of the abdominals is delivered to further activate the fiery

Prana. *Kapalabhati* improves digestion as well. A variation that I use is placing the index and middle fingers of both hands on the navel and pressing it vigorously while exhaling.

Bhastrika (bellows breath) often uses *kapalabhati* as a warm-up. Then one closes the left nostril with the little and ring finger of the right hand. In a comfortable position (seated or standing), one breathes in and out via the right nostril continuously and forcefully. A set of close to a dozen repetitions are performed. The last inhalation should be even deeper than before, with retention of air as long as possible until one begins to sense a slight suffocation. One immediately exhales via the left nostril while keeping the right pinched with the right thumb. One can add another round of *bhastrika*, reversing the nostrils. This kind of breathing is very effective in clearing mucus and all sorts of congestion from the head sinuses and the chest region. It also builds up digestive powers and tends to reduce one's fat weight (it could be employed in the process of making a weight for a contest).

Ujjayi (breath that leads to victory) involves inhalation via both nostrils while keeping the glottis slightly closed. Narrowing the glottis upon inhalation will cause a sound to be made. Next, one retains the air for as long as comfortable while keeping the chin locked and pinching both nostrils closed. What follows is a left-nostril exhalation that is twice as long as one's inhalation. *Ujjayi* breathing is a gentle way to increase one's fire energy and yet stay grounded in one's practice while strengthening one's diaphragm. It is particularly recommended for vata and pitta types who might be thrown off-balance by the more intense forms of breathing. A set of ten to twelve breaths is recommended.

In *surya bhedana* (sun-piercing breath), one inhales through right nostril (closing the left) and retains air until slight perspiration and a mild feeling of suffocation. After that, air is exhaled through the left nostril. A repetition of five to seven times should be sufficient. *Surya bhedana* is very effective in neutralizing and warding off various types of common cold.

Breathing According to the Five Types of Chi

After reading the section on the five types of Chi you may be asking yourself, "Which Pranas do I need to optimize for my functioning or for my combative art? How?" The answer to this question partially lies in the fact that martial artists will mostly need to develop Vyana Vayu, and there is a specific breathing technique to enhance it. The second part of the answer is that everyone needs the other types of Chi in the right proportions for their unique body type. For example, without Prana Vayu, there is no question of expanding and expressing oneself through Udana Vayu. Without Apana Vayu, we will not be able to eliminate any unusable, harmful elements—such as toxic wastes—from the system, and they will back up into our system, causing much harm on both the mental and physical levels. Thus, you can practice all five types of breathing daily or focus on certain ones, knowing well your weaknesses. You focus on certain types of pranayama by performing more Vayu-specific inhalations, retentions, and exhalations. With this in view, we will present five types of breathing for developing five specific types of Chi.

Prana Vayu. This is enhanced by deep inhalation of fresh air with one or both nostrils.[9] One can visualize drawing the energy from above into the nostrils and head, especially into the point between the eyebrows (known as the third eye). Visualization or imagery is essential to many breathing techniques, as it directs and grounds our flimsy mind during that time. Thus, it allows for energizing the mind and letting it carry and deliver the Prana to the various body parts.

---

[9] Alternate-nostril breathing is applicable here. You can first do the right-nostril breathing (*surya bhedana*), and thus focus on one side of the head, and then do the left nostril.

For my pranayama practice, I usually either stand in the doorway (when it's colder and windier) or step out into the backyard and watch the rising sun or morning sun. (Frawley, *Yoga and Ayurveda*, 251) I draw and absorb the radiant sunlight into my head, brain, mind, or the third eye. During inner retention, one can hold the energy in the third eye. One tries visualizing either a ball of light or a flame and how it is distributed to the rest of the body and its senses. It is important to note here that one can channel the Pranic energy to the location of their choice and thus aid in energizing, healing, and rejuvenating it.

Important herbs, Ayurvedic and otherwise, that help increase Prana Vayu are those that induce sweating (diaphoretics), open your sinuses, and stimulate the mind and senses, such as shilajit, eucalyptus, cinnamon, clove, pippali, sage, mint, thyme, and calamus. (190–91)

Udana Vayu. Contrary to most types of pranayama, where one is supposed to inhale through the nose, here one is advised to take a deep breath with the mouth and bring energy into the throat region. As one retains the breath, they try to focus the mind on holding the energy in the throat area. Next, one exhales through the mouth, visualizing that their energy rises like a ball of flame or light and envelops everything they see in front of them and even everything that they cannot see but that could potentially be on the horizon. When one practices Udana Vayu breath, they can help alleviate any weaknesses of the vocal chords and increase the strength of their voice. (252) A stronger warrior yell, *kiai*, is another benefit of this practice. A more powerful *kiai* energizes one even more, adds confidence, allows for expressing their spirit, and can shake up their opponent's equilibrium.

Some herbs, Ayurvedic and otherwise, that enhance Udana Vayu are spicy, astringent ones that strengthen the voice and reduce cough, such as haritaki, peppermint, vasa, cherry bark, licorice, calamus, elecampane, lobelia, and bayberry. (191)

Vyana Vayu. This breath resides mostly in the heart, but it saturates the entire physical body outwardly. Vyana Vayu pranayama should be done while standing. Upon taking a deep breath, one should extend the arms widely and fill the lungs and heart with Prana. During retention, one should still keep the arms open and visualize the energy traveling from the heart through one's arteries and through the whole body to one's limbs. As with the Udana Vayu pranayama, one can also include the external environment in this visualization. (252–53) I usually include the externals, like the trees and sky and even the gym I work at (at the end of retention). When exhaling, one should complete the channeling of energy to the limbs and the externals and return one's Prana back to the heart. One could see the Vyana Prana as orange in color. Practicing Vyana Vayu pranayama helps alleviate all sorts of circulatory and musculoskeletal impairments, such as asthma and arthritis. (253)

As for herbal supplementation for Vyana Vayu, we can consider spicy and bitter herbs that assist our circulation through the heart, blood, and musculoskeletal system, such as arjuna, angelica, guggul, kava kava, saffron, turmeric, guduchi, and Siberian ginseng. (191)

Samana Vayu. This is the breath in the belly. Samana Vayu pranayama balances one's physical and subtle (mind, intelligence) energies and helps alleviate any digestive problems. It is very good to practice if one experiences low appetite and does not absorb their food. As one inhales, they try to imagine the universal Prana traveling to their body from all corners of the universe. As one breathes in deeply, they attempt to direct the breath from the nostrils and head into their belly, igniting the digestive fire. One can visualize the stomach to be full of glowing rocks of coal that just need to be supplied air before they ignite. Upon holding, one imagines the fire blazing in their stomach. And when exhaling, one lets the breath travel and connect that concentrated fire with the rest of their body parts, including the mind. (253–54)

Ayurvedic supplements that are helpful in building up Samana Vayu are spicy and assist in nutrient absorption via the small intestine, such as cardamom, fennel, cayenne, ginger, mustard, cumin, basil, trikatu, nutmeg, and black pepper. (191)

Apana Vayu. This type of breathing will concentrate one's energy at the base of the spine. One takes a deep breath and directs it down to the root of spinal column. Practitioners can visualize themselves as a massive, heavy, and stable mountain connected to the Earth. One retains their breath in that region. Upon exhalation, one sends all the mental and physical toxins into the ground. One visualizes a deep-blue or blown color of the toxic energies leaving their system in the form of a stream intertwined with lightning flashes like a thunderbolt dispersing its energy into the ground. One may not need to imagine the sound. (254) When I perform pranayama for the Apana Vayu, I usually just hear my own concentrated breath pushing out the toxins (such as negative emotions, feelings, and attachments) and positive emotions (such as the happiness from my promotion at work, last night's birthday party, or a victorious sparring match).

It is helpful to exhale through the mouth here while tightening up the glottis to expel the toxins more rapidly and powerfully from the system. One should exhale as much air as possible and hardly leave anything in the gut. The outer retention is important here, and one should extend up to a slight feeling of suffocation. During outer retention, one should sense that all the toxins are gone, and one should stay in a detached mental state, having given up all negativities and positivities (see examples above). After that, one should inhale deeply, replenishing the Prana through Prana Vayu. Apana Vayu pranayama aids in the reproductive and excretory functions of the body and enhances one's immunity.

Herbal supplements and plants to try here are mild laxatives that aid in absorption of Prana via the large intestine, such as triphala, haritaki, psyllium, flax seed, castor oil, aloe vera, asafetida (hing), and hingvashtaka. (191)

Mudras and Their Usage in Combination with Breathing Techniques

"Gesture" or "seal" is the Sanskrit meaning of the word *mudra*. Mudras are often performed with both hands simultaneously, and they facilitate a more optimal energy flow in our bodies. We can call them, for our purposes, the asanas for the hands.

As you may recall from chapter I, "Ayurvedic Background," five elements—earth, water, fire, air, and ether—make up your body and the whole world. Your five fingers represent these five elements. The thumb conducts the fire element and the type of Chi known as Prana Vayu (the main Prana). The index finger conducts the air element and the type of Chi known as Udana Vayu. The middle finger conducts the ether element, and it relates to the type of Chi known as Vyana Vayu. The ring finger conducts the earth element, and it relates to Samana Vayu. The pinky conducts the water element and Apana Vayu. Bringing the thumb together with a finger will balance the element represented by that finger. For example, the joining of the thumb and the index finger will balance the air element. The thumb and index finger are often used in conjunction in healing massages. The joining of your thumb and middle finger will balance the ether element, and so on and so forth. The palm of your hand conducts all five types of Chi in combination.

When you sense that some of the elements in the combined forms of vata (air, ether), pitta (fire, air), or kapha (water, earth) are tending toward imbalance or are already out of balance, you may use the mudras in combination with other balancing technologies such as pranayama to speed up the recovery of your natural harmony. I personally use the mudras especially during breathing practice, after performing the asanas, and during mentally stressful moments.

There are many mudra hand positions, but the Prana, Vayu and Prithvi ones can be especially useful to martial artists. They are described as follows.

Prana Mudra. The Prana mudra energizes your body, strengthens the immune system, and boosts lethargic mood, thus diminishing post-workout fatigue. The earth and water elements will be brought into balance, as will the Samana and Apana Vayus. A workout—because of movement, exertion, and sweating—initially diminishes the earth, water, and fire elements in the body. In physiology, this is known as catabolism. Catabolic function is quite natural, but it must be reoriented into an anabolic function, or rebuilding. Hence, the diminished elements will start increasing again after being connected to the thumb, the Prana Vayu conductor.

One may assume a standing or seated position with their back straight. One touches the tips of their ring and pinky finger to the thumb. One performs the same technique with the other hand at the same time. The index and middle finger point out straight, and the palms are directed upward to the sky. One can practice the Prana mudra even for 30 minutes. I personally combine it with breathing that lasts five minutes or so. It can be practiced intermittently throughout the day, a few minutes or moments at a time.

Vayu Mudra. The Vayu mudra balances the air element in the body and the Prana known as Udana Vayu. During a heavy workout, one will deplete the outgoing Prana and the joints. Also, the air circulation tends to go upward rather then downward, and the downward movement needs to be reestablished. One joins the tips of both of their index fingers to the base of their thumbs. The index finger will be curved and the remaining fingers straight. One directs the palms of their hands downward to facilitate downward air flow. This is practiced in a standing or seated position for up to 15 minutes.

Prithvi Mudra. This particular mudra restores strength in the body by increasing the earth element and the Samana

Vayu. It draws the energy within after it has been expanded outward in an intense workout, thus alleviating post-workout fatigue. While standing or sitting with the spine erect, one touches the tip of the ring finger of each hand to the tip of the thumb. One positions the palms of their hands upward close to their sides. The Prithvi mudra is practiced for up to 10 minutes.

In addition to the few mudras described above, it is important to note that the holding of ones half-folded hands (fingers touching), palms facing up, will orient more of the five Pranas to the head to increase mental energy, whereas holding the hands palms down will transport them down and calm one down.

Breathing Techniques in Traditional Karate[10]

There are essentially three types of breathing used in the practice of karate that come under the term *ibuki* (Japanese for "breath"): front loud-breath *ibuki*, front silent-breath *ibuki*, and back silent-breath *ibuki*. All of them focus on regenerating Ki (Chi) after or during karate sessions and are performed in a standing position,

---

[10] Adapted from Mas Oyama, *Complete Karate Course*, 82–85.

usually in the order listed below. They are supposed to be practiced several times a day, so they may not be limited to karate practice alone, although we can practice karate more than once a day.[11] At our dojo, we practiced them at the end of the session, when the body was fully stretched, exercised, and tired, which made the breathing exercises more effective. I will briefly describe them below.

Front loud breath. From a neutral stance, hands by the hips, one starts by making tight fists. One inhales silently and slowly while bringing the fists up and crossing them at sides of the neck. At that time the fingers should be tight but extended. The focus here is on a very full inhalation that is directed inside the lower abdominal muscles. One is trying to channel Ki from outside into the stomach. Once the stomach, lungs, and head are maximally full of air, there is a mini retention followed by a noisy exhalation through a partially closed glottis and an open mouth. The lips could be curled, as if one wants to blow candles, while uncrossing the arms and making fists again. One should attempt to force the air out as much as possible using the lower abdominals. At the end of the exhalation, all the muscles in the body should be contracted strongly, and the mind should be

---

[11] I still vividly remember the karate camp I went to where we practiced three times daily, each workout over one hour long so that breathing exercises were done more than once.

focused on the lower abdominals (extra contraction over there).

The goal of this loud and strong type of breathing is not only to exercise the abdominal muscles and lungs but also to seize a lot of Ki and channel it down to the point below the navel. The long and powerful exhalation results in a cleansing action for the physical and subtle body (mind, intelligence).[12] In our dojo we used to prolong the exhalation in a series of final abdominal contractions as if to expel any remaining air. It looked like one was choking and was trying to cough up a piece of food. A slight feeling of suffocation might occur only to be followed by a very deep inhalation.

Front silent breath. One begins with arms stretched out in front of them (but not locked). One turns the palms of their hands upward and begins to inhale quietly while bringing both hands to the chest. From there, one begins lowering the hands slowly, exhaling quietly through the nose or mouth while turning the palms of the hands down. This is repeated as necessary. The focus here is on absorbing external Ki and distributing it throughout the body (Vyana Vayu). We practiced the front silent breath at the end of an intense karate session.

---

[12] It is known in yoga practice that the images one receives from the external world should be properly "digested" by the intelligence. Anything undigested creates blockages on the subtle level. Toward the end of the exhalation portion and also during outer retention of breath, one eliminates these from the system.

Back silent breath. One begins with their arms and hands down. One bends their elbows slightly, with their palms up so they face forward and away from oneself. While inhaling slowly, one brings the hands to chest level. At the top of such a deep inhalation, one retains, contracts all the muscles (especially the elbows, legs, and middle fingers), turns the palms down, and begins extending the hands forward. It should look like one is thrusting the contracted fingers of their hands at the opponent. This portion is done in slow motion while holding the breath.[13] The focus of total muscle tension should switch to the lower abdomen, sides, and still fingertips. Once the arms and hands are extended fully (without lockout), one should exhale, relax, and return the hands to original palm up position. The focus here is on distributing Ki (Samana and Vyana Vayus) to the important limbs of the body that are used in punching, kicking, and defending.

Each of these types of breathing can be repeated numerous times before the *karateka* (one who practices the art of karate) moves on to the next type. Thus, one could perform the front loud breath three times, the front silent breath four times, and the back silent breath three times.

---

[13] In our dojo we did this portion very quickly by actually performing a palm / finger thrust while retaining the breath.

Neti Pot

The essential item in maintaining a high level of Prana Vayu and being able to absorb it properly is daily cleansing of the nasal passages. Optimizing the function of the nostrils is accomplished through the neti pot, which purifies the sinuses. The neti pot is a special pot made specifically for this purpose, and it is used by yoga practitioners. The neti pot procedure is best done before your morning yoga practice and breathing exercises, and it takes only a few minutes.

Optionally, obtain baby bottle and cut off the top with scissors. Put a pinch or two of Himalayan salt or other high-quality salt in that bottle. Pour about four to eight ounces of potable and lukewarm water in it. Tilt your head back and tilt the bottle so that the water starts flowing into the right nostril.

Once a portion of water is in the nostril, make sure it goes all the way up while you contract your throat so as not to swallow the water. Hold for a few seconds. The muscle action here is identical to when you gargle salted water to alleviate a sore throat. Next, while holding the chin up, tilt your head sideways to the left so that the water penetrates deeper and crosses into the left nostril. Then tilt your head down so that the water pours out of the left nostril. Repeat the steps once or twice more and reverse to do the same with the left nostril. When you have water left, just use it up, alternating between the nostrils. You should be able to use up the full eight-ounce bottle. Have a piece of cloth ready for impurities that come out, and feel free to blow your nose every time you switch nostrils.

You will feel a great difference in the quality of your breathing. It is best to do your alternate-nostril breathing immediately after using the neti pot. Then proceed to yoga asanas. Then, do your pranayama breathing routine.

Three Levels of Energy Centers

Mind and intelligence (subtle body) and the self (spiritual body) are linked to the gross body via the chakras, nadis, and marmas. Chakras, the least tangible of the three, are the energy centers of the subtle body positioned along the spinal column. The nadis are the subtle channels that extend and travel from the chakras to many points on the physical body and charge the fourteen physiological systems (see the "Optimum Amount of Tension in the Systems" section in chapter V). They are not truly physical nerves but rather perceptible energy flows. Finally, marmas, which we will focus on in this chapter, are actual physical pressure points of high sensitivity that unfold from the nadis. They function as energy distributors of vital Prana from the chakras and the nadis to the whole body. (Frawley, *Ayurveda and Marma Therapy*, 41–42)

Marma Points in the Martial Arts[14]

It is my intention here to briefly mention a few of the vital marma points and when and how to stimulate them so as to aid in one's combative practice. Martial artists, athletes, and their coaches should be familiar with such natural energy stimulants. Understanding the value of marma points will no doubt enhance any type of martial arts and warrior practices, be they beginner or advanced.

The secret knowledge of vital points, pressure points, has been a part of both the medical and martial arts traditions for thousands of years. In ancient medical fields such as Ayurveda or Traditional Chinese Medicine, this knowledge has served as a healing tool to directly harmonize the patient's energy, life force, in the physical body. The physical points on the body were, so to speak, entrances into a person's deeper layer of armor, the subtle armor, and could therefore adjust its potencies. In the traditional martial arts such as karate or kalaripayit, marma points (*kyusho* in Japanese) have been used to effectively disable aggressors without using much force. A warrior in knowledge of such points was able to manipulate the points and alter the functioning of his/ her own body. In fact, the ancient warrior code of conduct stressed the development of personal power with qualities of courage, self-discipline, determination, etc. and, therefore, a good control over one's Prana.

---

[14] Adapted from Frawley, *Ayurveda and Marma Therapy*, 9.

The marmas constitute centers for Prana, and they vary in size, from very small to quite large. There are approximately 108 of them categorized into six main regions: the head, neck, heart, bladder, endocrine system, and reproductive system. Their function is like that of power switches that either turn Prana on or off, or up and down. They are intimately related to nadis and chakras. Marmas control communication and energy exchange between one's physical body and subtle body (mind, ego, intelligence, and corollary emotions and moods). Thus, when properly triggered, marmas can restore the optimal connection between them.

It is worth mentioning that special mantras may be recited during or after one's yoga/stretching practice to enhance emotional power, or the subtle armor. When you perform your mantra meditation properly according to your body type and mental constitution, then you will become more aware of how well or not the energy flows through the marmas. One such mantra is found in the ancient *Srimad-Bhagavatam* scripture composed of 18,000 Sanskrit verses, in the chapter where the king of heaven, Indra, becomes victorious over the soldiers of the demons. (SB, 6.8) A very abbreviated version of it is as follows:

> *"Please explain to me that Narayana armor, by which King Indra achieved success in battle, conquering the enemies who were endeavoring to kill him."*

"If some form of fear arrives, one should first wash his hands and legs clean and then chant this mantra:

"om apavitrah pavitro va
sarvavastham gato 'pi va
yah smaret pundarikaksham
sa bahyabhayantarah shucih
sri-vishnu sri-vishnu sri-vishnu

"Thus, in the following manner, he should bind himself with the Narayana coat of armor. First, chant the mantra om namo narayanaya, then om namo bhagavate vasudevaya, then om vishnave namaha. After finishing this chanting, one should think himself qualitatively one with the Supreme Personality of Godhead, who is full in six opulences and is worthy to be meditated upon. Then one should chant the following protective prayer, the Narayana-kavacha:

"The Supreme Lord, who sits on the back of the bird Garuda, touching him with his lotus feet, holds eight weapons—the conchshell, disc, shield, club, arrows, bow, and ropes. O Indra, this mystic armor related to Lord Narayana has been described by me to you. By putting on this protective covering, you will certainly be able to conquer the leaders of the demons."

In the ancient martial arts of India, marmas were related to the use of body armor (*varma* in Sanskrit). The armor was made to protect the sensitive points on the warrior's body. For example, in the classic epic *Mahabharata*, in which a great world war occurs, there are numerous mentions of protective coverings for the vital points of elephants, horses, and soldiers.

Today, South India still has a very complete and original system of martial arts called kalaripayit, of which the highest form is called *marma adi*. In *marma adi*, the knowledge of vital points is essential. It is known that the healing art of *varma chikitsa* (marma therapy) originates from *marma adi*.

As you may remember from the section on traditional Ashtanga yoga, one of its preliminary tenets was the practice of *ahimsa*, nonviolence, so yoga practitioners and Buddhist monks were not allowed to carry and use weapons. Forms of empty-hand combat were taught to them as needed. Master Bodhidharma, who is noted for bringing Zen meditation and combative arts to China, came from a well-reputed yoga center in Kanchipuram, South India. Therefore, it is quite probable that Chinese medicine has used some aspects of Indian marma therapy, as evidenced by the similarities between acupuncture and marma therapy.

Marmas in the head and neck are most numerous because the head has the most openings that connect us to the external world. Through these openings we draw Prana to our body-mind system. As marmas in the head are small, acupressure would work better than massage. I will mention only five of them here. As you go through these marma points, it may be helpful to revisit the "Five Types of Chi" section in chapter IV.

The *phana* (a serpent's hood) is located on the side of the nostrils at the base of the nose and nasal openings on the facial artery and vein. More points are found along the bridge of the nose going all the way up to the eye sockets. This important energy point controls important Prana channels that go to the brain, the nasal passages, and the sinuses, and it is likely the most essential marma point for the purpose of pranayama. One can use a strong circular motion for a few minutes at those points or along the side of the nose using the index finger. In addition, peppermint, eucalyptus, or camphor oil can be placed below the nasal openings (or diffused in the room) to aid in stimulating the marmas. (Frawley, *Ayurveda and Marma Therapy*, 184–86) I find stimulating this marma particularly helpful before a cardio workout, after the neti pot procedure or before the alternate-nostril breathing that precedes my morning stretches. It neutralizes the morning congestion from the nose and lungs, optimizing our capacity to take in air and, therefore, oxygen. It especially boosts aerobic performance.

The *utkshepa* (what is cast upward) is located behind the upper part of each ear's helix, on the internal carotid arteries. It is a crucial point to control the energy of vata in the form of Apana Vayu and, therefore, the mind. To calm down the mind before or after a tough competition bout, one or one's coach can use gentle circular motions with fingers or thumbs. Calming essential oils such as sandalwood or valerian can be diffused or applied topically to the location as well for enhanced effect. Massage oils such as almond or sesame can be rubbed on this marma. (195–96)

The *avarta* (calamity, a point of high sensitivity) is located in the upper part of the orbital cavity (eye socket), in the middle of each eyebrow, on the supraorbital arteries. For improving one's general energy and equilibrium in the form of Prana Vayu, one can use the fingers and specifically the middle finger to gently massage the spot. Massage oils such as sesame or almond can be used to magnify the effect. Essential oils such as peppermint, eucalyptus, or camphor can be used to stimulate Prana going to the head and the body in general. Caution should be taken not to get any of the aromatic oils into the eyes. (197–98)

The *shringataka* (a point where four roads meet) is located internally on the soft palate, but the corresponding external point will work. The external corresponding region is found between the upper border of the cheek bone and the base of the nose (infraorbital foramen). Yogis understand this point as a meeting place of energies of the tongue, nose, eyes, and ears, all of which are essential to our optimal functioning. This crucial point controls Prana Vayu and the finer, subtle forms of kapha (water and earth elements of the physical body). The *shringataka* is therefore used mainly to rejuvenate one's body-mind system after a tough workout or tough day at work. One should gently massage the point with almond or sesame oil. To maximize the powers of one's senses, one should use essential oils such as frankincense, calamus, myrrh, or peppermint. The internal point can be stimulated by sucking on spicy herbs like cloves and holding the herbs at the back of one's mouth. (199–200)

The *sthapani* (that which gives support) is found between the eyebrows, where, according to yoga science, lies the third eye.[15] The *sthapani* is a very important point of mind and sense control. The point closer to the middle of the forehead, according to other yoga experts, facilitates overcoming one's mind, whereas the point between the eyebrows makes the control of one's senses easier. If a martial artist wants to

---

[15] This is a focal point in meditation (*dhyana*) in the Eightfold Yoga System of Ashtanga. By placing attention there, one can develop a great concentration and rediscover one's latent higher powers of perception.

focus and pacify the mind between an important bout, then he/she should use a strong circular motion for a few minutes to achieve the desired effect. One should use almond or sesame oil when pressing or massaging the point and aromatic oils such as peppermint, camphor, etc. to release stress accumulated in the mind and senses. (201–2)

Marmas in the arms and hands contain energy points that are very important for martial artists and athletes because they perform a lot of physical tasks with arms and hands. As previously mentioned, the Vyana Vayu is the kind of Prana directly responsible for outward momentum of energy (expressive force). Due to the symmetry of our physical bodies, the marmas on the arms contain a point on each side of the body. The right-side marmas promote the increase of heat (stimulate them before working out), whereas the left-side marmas promote cooling of the body (stimulate them after a workout/rejuvenation).

The *kshipra* (immediately effective) is located between the thumb and index finger on both sides of the hand (between the first and second metacarpal bones). The *kshipra* marma controls the respiratory system, heart, lungs, and both Prana and Vyana Vayus. Its stimulation is, therefore, useful before doing anaerobic and aerobic workouts. One should use a strong circular motion on the spot for a few minutes or just press and hold the point. It will definitely help one with overall circulation of blood throughout the body. Essential oils such as cinnamon, sage, or eucalyptus can be used to further stimulate the energy and relieve pain in the limbs. (96–97)

The *talahridaya* (center of the surface) is found in the center of the palm and plays an important role in energy circulation of the whole body, especially function of the respiratory system, heart, and lungs. By stimulating *talahridaya* marmas, one can optimize Vyana Vayu (the circulating Prana) in the area above the navel. (98–99) It is worth mentioning here that the left and right arms' combative or purely physical performance will be enhanced, especially before punching combination drills. One can use strong circular motions to massage the point and can use eucalyptus, cinnamon, or camphor.

The *manibandha* (bracelet) is situated lateral to the center of the wrist joint and also on the opposite side (back of wrist). By stimulating this point, the skeletal system is strengthened (joint lubrication), the movement of hands improved, and Vyana Vayu, or the peripheral circulating Prana, increased. The martial arts practitioner can massage the *manibandha* point with moderate strength using either sesame or almond oil to strengthen the joints. Essential oils such as wintergreen, birch, myrrh, or angelica can be used to relieve joint pain and swelling after a heavy sparring practice. (104–5)

The *bahvi* (that which relates to the arm) is located in the upper arm, close to the brachial artery and vein on the biceps and triceps muscles. By strongly massaging the point in a circular way for a few minutes, a martial arts practitioner can enhance Vyana Vayu (peripheral circulating Prana) and optimal growth of bodily tissue (skin, muscle, bone, etc.). Oils that can be used are sesame, almond, and mustard seed. Essential oils that are used to increase Vyana Vayu here are cinnamon and ginger. (112–13)

The *lohitaksha* (red-jointed) is situated at the center of each armpit of each shoulder. The axillary artery has its passage there. This marma point is responsible, among other functions, for the control of Vyana Vayu, specifically to the legs. (114–15) It is a smart idea to stimulate it before a heavy-duty leg drill or a workout that involves any sort of running. Using essential oils such as eucalyptus, cinnamon, or peppermint on the location will certainly magnify the effect.

The *kakshadhara* (that which upholds the flanks) is located near the top of the shoulder joint on each arm, between the pectoralis major and minor (chest muscles), or the shoulder girdle's lateral edge of the tip of the coracoid process. This marma point governs the muscular system of your body, specifically the shoulders. Bodily posture and Vyana Vayu also come under its command. (116–17) Because of the above, *kakshadhara* is a great point for athletes and martial artists to stimulate via massage or acupressure. Before a training session, a warrior can sharpen his/her Vyana Vayu for punching, kicking, etc. They can use essential oils such as eucalyptus, cinnamon, and myrrh on the spot. After a heavy-duty training, one can release muscular tension from the whole body and use sesame oil.

Marma points of the lower body are the same in number and name as those in the upper body because they mirror one another. Legs and feet have many points to receive vital Prana from the ground and to express our Prana in such activities like running, jumping, and kicking. Like the marmas in the upper body, the lower body marmas have two points, one on each leg and foot. Stimulation of the left-side marmas has more of a cooling action whereas stimulation of the right-side marmas heats up the body (increasing metabolism, increasing digestion, etc.).

The *kshipra* (immediately effective) is found between the big and first toe and controls the respiratory system (heart and lungs in general). It is good to use strong circular movement on this spot to induce a good flow of Prana in the lower body. (120–21)

Martial artists and athletes who use their lower limbs extensively can benefit from stimulating this point. The essential oils used for opening up energy flow in the lungs (e.g., clearing the lungs) should be eucalyptus, camphor, and cinnamon.

The *talahridaya* (center of the surface) is found in the upper center of the sole, below the base of the third toe of each foot. This important point controls the respiratory system and the feet as well. The *talahridaya* marma restores and optimizes the circulating Prana (Vyana Vayu) in the lower body and the area below the navel, particularly the feet. (122–23) It stabilizes the earth element in the body, so it is especially important for vatas and pittas to frequently massage. Those body types will tend to have excessive air, ether, and fire elements in their systems due to both their nature and intense training. The *talahridaya* also keeps the downward moving Prana in balance (Apana Vayu). One can use a strong circular motion for a few minutes until one feels the energy released and balanced again. Sesame or almond oils can be used to strengthen the feet and calm down the mind. To improve circulation in the lower body, one can use essential oils such as juniper, garlic, and cedar.

The *gulpha* (ankle joint) is located on the inside of the ankle joint of each leg and just below the round ankle bone. This particular marma point controls the growth of bones, maintenance of fat tissue, lubrication of joints, the circulating Prana (Vyana Vayu), and the movement of your feet. (128–29) Martial artists and athletes who are in the mesocycle of leaning out can use this point to drop body fat by applying a gentle circular motion for a few minutes. Mustard oil and peppermint or camphor essential oils can be used to that effect. Stimulating that area will enhance footwork patterns worked by various athletes.

The *lohitaksha* (red-jointed) is situated on the lower frontal area of the hip joint of each leg, specifically over the femoral artery and nerve, over the psoas major muscle. This marma location is in charge of both Vyana and Apana Vayus, which are the peripheral and downward moving Prana. (138–39) The *lohitaksha* specifically delivers energy to the legs and as such is very important to athletes of all sorts and specifically martial artists. For improvement in circulation, one can use sesame oil or essential oils such as myrrh and cinnamon.

Marmas on the front of the body (abdominals, chest) are lesser in number but nonetheless important. They shelter the main vital organs.

The *nabhi* (navel) is found on and around the navel and controls the digestive and circulatory systems. It is the major energy center for exertion and digestion, the overall fire energy (pitta) in the body (148–49), hence it is of utmost importance for both athletes or whoever has a very physical type of work (e.g., construction worker). One can massage the area with circular motions around the belly button for a few minutes. This is the main area for reducing the fire energy, be it excessive aggressiveness, anger, fever, etc. Sesame or almond oils can be used for stress relief for vatas or kaphas. For pitta-dominant warriors, coconut oil would be a better choice. Meditation on this marma point can help balance all five types of Chi and improve physical strength (see "Three Levels of Energy Centers" in this chapter). Pressing this point quickly and deeply (like a mini CPR) on the exhalation portion of breathing practice will improve metabolism. It is a good idea to combine a five-minute Samana Vayu breathing with a *nabhi* marma massage session to get the most results out of one's massage.

The *hridaya* (heart) is situated in the heart region in the middle of the sternum and controls the circulatory system, overall strength, and immunity. As such, the *hridaya* marma affects mental power, Vyana Vayu, and Prana Vayu. Gentle massage of this area with sesame oil has a calming effect and helps relieve stress and any negative emotions. Sandalwood essential oil can be used to rid excessive aggressiveness and hyperactivity when applied to the *hridaya* marma. (88–91)

Sometimes we complete our workouts late in the day and such emotions will get in the way of our rest. This way we can get a sounder sleep for the upcoming day. At other times, after tough training days, a warrior may feel some laziness and lethargy kicking in, and our tight training schedule may call for getting up very early, depriving us of some sleep. During such times, it is good to apply mustard oil, eucalyptus, or ginger essential oil with somewhat stronger circular movements on the spot to improve Vyana, the power of circulation, and remove stagnation.

The *stanarohita* (upper region of the chest) is located above the nipples and a little to the center of the chest, on the ends of the pectoral muscle. It controls both the muscular and nervous systems along with the Prana and Vyana types of Chi. Application of sesame oil with strong circular motions will calm the emotions, while essential oils like valerian, juniper, basil, and sage will improve circulation of Prana in the muscles and brain. (155–56)

The *apalapa* (unguarded) is located in the armpit region in the area above and around the subclavian artery and vein, a little below the *kakshadhara* marma point (see above). The *apalapa* is in control of the nerve flow to the arms and therefore peripheral circulation to the arms, or Vyana Vayu. (157–58) A martial artist can stimulate it to relieve muscular and nervous tension in the shoulder, upper back, and neck area after intense punching drills. Good oils to use for tuning down the nervous system are almond and sesame, while basil and valerian can be used to release muscle tension.

Vital points in the hips are an important place of accumulation of water and earth elements. They are of importance to vatas and pittas who would like to gain weight and/or stabilize their heightened and jumpy levels of energy. The upper back (shoulder area) is a place of Prana accumulation because it is connected to the heart and lungs.

The *katikataruna* (that which rises from the hip) is located at each hip joint on the back side of the body and supports bones and the skeletal system in general. It greatly relieves the accumulated powers of vata (air and ether) and is thus important for vatas to stimulate. (162–63) A martial artist involved in a lot of lower body work such as kicking, jumping, and pushing (which draws power from the ground) will benefit by using a strong circular motion here, for it will relieve tension in the pelvic and hip area and improve bone strength. Essential oils recommended for repairing and strengthening bones are camphor, wintergreen, and myrrh. One can also use sesame or almond oils.

The *brihati* (wide or large) is found below each lower side of the scapula, or shoulder blade, and is in charge Vyana Vayu (circulating Prana) in the arms. Stimulating these points will augment one's qualities of courage and determination, which are the refined qualities of fire element in the body. When one applies a strong circular massage to the area, one can relieve tension from the areas of the shoulders and heart. Sesame oil is good, and essential oils such as sandalwood are used. It is important to note that one can achieve an enhanced or more balanced effect by stimulating both the *brihati* and *hridaya* marmas on opposite side of body (see above). (170–71)

The *amshaphalaka* (shoulder blade) is found on each shoulder blade, just above the *brihati*, at the level of cervical vertebrae—five through seven and the first thoracic, overlaying portions of the rhomboid and trapezius muscles. This important marma supports the respiratory system and the Prana and Vyana Vayus. To unlock the Prana and Vyana Vayus in the arms and lungs, one simply uses a strong circular movement for a few minutes. Useful essential oils are peppermint, eucalyptus, and camphor. (172–73) It is especially important to stimulate this marma point for a combat athlete who uses a lot of upper-body work (punches, takedowns, blocks, etc.).

Chapter V

Spiritual Armor:

Mantras of Ancient Masters

Yogic Mantra—Polishing the Mirror of the Mind

Mantra, sound that liberates the mind from ordinary thought processes, has been recorded in ancient yoga books and practiced for thousands of years by yogis, ancient physicians, and ancient warriors such as the *maharathas* or *atirathas*.[16] Mantras exist in the original language of humankind, or Sanskrit, and each mantra is connected to a specific point on the body. Along with herbs to heal the body, mantra repetition has been used in Ayurveda to heal the mind of patients (*mantra chikitsha*). After all, sound is the primeval form of all energy.

---

[16] These are the warriors who, according to the ancient text *Mahabharata*, could fight 1,000 to 10,000 ordinary soldiers at a time primarily by being able to utter secret sound vibrations.

Mantras can be monosyllabic such as *om*, or they can be verse, such as *om namo bhagavate vasudevaya*. Their lengths vary from just one syllable to even hundreds or thousands. Different mantras can be recommended to people in the mode of goodness, passion, and ignorance. They are usually prescribed to one by one's teacher, or guru. Mantras consist of three parts: *bindu* (latent potency residing in the sound), *nada* (external sound of the mantra that everyone can hear), and *bija* (seed or goal of the mantra attained by the chanter).

Mantras are closely related to marmas, or sensitive energy points on the body (see section above). By repeating mantra sound vibrations, a martial artist, or anybody, for that matter, will release more Prana and empower the physical body and mind for more optimal functioning. Furthermore, the chanted mantras possess a protective function, *kavacha* in Sanskrit, that can guard the vital marmas on the warrior's body.

As amazing as it seems, they do require of us a consistent practice to ensure results, under the keen eye of one's qualified teacher.[17] Mantra repetition has been used in various types of yoga for ascending to higher

---

[17] According to the *Vedas*, or the ancient scriptures of knowledge, one must approach a spiritual master to receive the spiritual vibration, or mantra, properly. Such spiritual disciplic successions of masters are known as a *parampara*. Otherwise, the effects of chanting mantras without proper guidance are unpredictable and even detrimental.

levels of consciousness/perception of reality.[18] Mantra has even earned its own form of yoga: mantra-yoga. The physical body has its exercises in the form of asanas. Similarly, the mind can be said to have its own set of exercises, the various mantras.

In 2015, there was a study presented in *Brain and Behavior* journal to the effect that a silent repetition of a nondescriptive word can have a profound physiological effect, such as lowered cortisol hormone levels (the hormone responsible for breakdown of tissues), decreased perception of workout-induced pain, enhanced cardiovascular endurance, improved mood, increased concentration, and lengthening of telomeres (which is linked to increased longevity).

Mantra is the best way for a warrior to enter and deeply explore the levels of his/her own Prana on a daily basis. Mantra meditation allows the warrior to keep the sharpest mind for determining the right action from moment to moment and deciding the right workout approach for the particular body type from day to day. Have you ever driven a car on three or four hours of

---

[18] As you may gather from the chapter on Ashtanga yoga, mantra meditation usually would follow the typical asana (physical postures) and pranayama (breathing exercises) practice. It would fall under the *dhyana* level but could also have its place anywhere between levels five and seven of Ashtanga, the reason being that after asana and pranayama pacify the mind, it can focus more steadily on a chosen object, be it a physical object of meditation or a sacred mantra sound. It can be frustrating to practice a mantra if one's mind is very flickering and hyperactive. Thus, mantra is a more esoteric (internal and secret) and advanced form of traditional Ashtanga yoga.

sleep while the cup of coffee that you had prepared stayed forgotten on the kitchen table? Yes, same here. That cup of coffee or green tea surely makes a difference when reading your car's control panel and observing the quickly moving world outside the window. Well, when you go about your day, do not forget your cup of coffee— your mantra meditation. You will enable yourself to discern your body's and mind's needs much better than without it. You will discern real need from flimsy desire.

Before you get started on any mantra presented here, you should know that such powerful mantras should be used only to further spiritual, mental, and physical healing of our bodies and the bodies of others, *not* to fulfill selfish desires or harm other living entities. This is a very important point to keep in mind. The power of mantra can be likened to the force of electricity. When you are a qualified electrician, you can work with the force of electricity and create wonders, but if you are not, then you can easily harm yourself and others. Therefore, without following the regulations given forth by the ancient yogis and sages, one will end up harming oneself in the long run and surely obtain adverse karmic reactions.[19]

---

[19] The universal law of karma is a vast and complex subject matter beyond the scope of this book. Suffice it to say that the proverbial adage "as you sow you shall reap" is extended to indicate and encompass the situation we are presently in as borne out of our previous existence and also its lasting effects beyond our present situation, shaping factors of our future existence.

In this chapter I will present a few of the original root sound vibrations with their specific effects on your psyche, as well as which body types benefit from specific mantras the most. I have been using the mantra tool myself for a long time with a noticeable effect on my consciousness. When you attempt your best to align the Prana according to the prescription in this book, you can enable yourself to chant the mantras properly.

Ram ("a" pronounced as in "father") is a powerful mantra for attracting the protective universal energy. Its effects include peace, inner strength, and improved immunity of the nervous system. At the external level, it will affect one's sleep quality. It is especially good for a vata body type with a vata mental predisposition. It can be visualized as brownish and/or reddish.

Hum (pronounced as "whom") is a potent mantra form neutralizing negative energies from other individuals, environmental pathogens, and one's own destructive emotions. At the external level, it affects one's digestive acid in a positive way.[20] On the internal level, it facilitates a better control over one's mental powers, such as those of perception. It is said to be the most important mantra for protecting vital marma points and can be visualized

---

[20] The action of an individual's hydrochloric acid is a very important indicator and predictor of health and ability to burn up accumulated toxins.

in a deep-blue color. (Frawley, *Ayurveda and Marma Therapy*, 54)

Om traditionally indicates the Absolute, or the totality of universal energies within and without the universe. Much like Prana Vayu, or the main Prana in the physical body, this special mantra is the foundation of all the processes in the body, from chemical to subtle (mental functioning, thought processes). *Om* helps our energies to ascend. It clears the mind and intelligence and facilitates healing forces of Prana that help in an individual's healing process (after sustaining any type of injury). Since it carries a solar energy, it can be imagined as golden.

Aim (pronounced "I'm") stimulates one's ability to focus, think rationally, and speak. It also boosts one's creativity by augmenting intelligence. When *aim* is chanted, it will assist an individual in coping with nervous problems and direct mental energy to a particular marma point for healing purposes. It holds the energy of wisdom and can be visualized as white.

Shrim (pronounced "shreem") is an important mantra for boosting general health, beauty, and prosperity. When chanted, it also nourishes the nervous system by projecting lunar energy. Just like the *som* mantra below, this one is very useful for combative athletes who train hard and therefore easily run into tissue depletion via overtraining to achieve their goals. It is a "recovery" mantra and can be visualized in a shade of light green, yellow, or orange.

Hrim (pronounced "hreem") is a great mantra for detoxification and cleansing. It provides the chanter with energy and happiness. *Hrim* will realign one's mental state and so is good to use after very important events that shake up one's psychological balance. *Hrim* is the main mantra of the divine mother, or feminine aspect of all universal energies, and can be seen as golden in color.

Krim (pronounced "cream") is excellent for all active people and especially athletes who use their bodies a lot. It affords one work capacity and power for efficient action. It is said that when you prepare medicine for yourself, or any food for that matter, the *krim* mantra will make the food or herbs improve their efficient action on your system. We can see it in our mind's eye as dark blue in color.

Klim (pronounced "kleem") is an interesting mantra to gain control over one's emotions. It is also good for increasing strength in general in the aspect of stability and balance. Thus, it is a very good sound vibration for those with vata natures. It is visualized as red in color.

Haum ("au" pronounced as in "owl") augments one's ability of personal transformation by increasing wisdom, power, and strength. Prana Vayu is greatly enhanced by chanting *haum*, as are subtle forms of fire (there are twelve). It is visualized as black in color.

Sham ("a" pronounced as in "gum") is a peace mantra that encourages satisfaction, calm, and a detached mood. It helps the chanter overcome disturbances of emotional and mental nature. The *sham* mantra works particularly well for pitta types, who are known for their fiery natures. It can be visualized as indigo in color.

Som ("o" pronounced as in "roam") is great for overall energy enhancement, happiness, and creativity. *Som* improves mental strength and strengthens the heart and nervous system. Warriors who work very hard by exerting their bodies in martial arts training, or any committed athletes, for that matter, will greatly benefit by chanting the *som* mantra and rejuvenating themselves. It can be visualized as white in color.

Mantras per Your Constitution

Vata mantras should be soft and calming. Vatas should not chant loud or long, to prevent their energy from being depleted. They can alternate the louder and silent chanting,[21] which is what I do in my meditation. When you wake up with your energy already low, begin chanting softer while listening to an audio recording of the same mantra. This will awaken your mind so that you can chant with more mindfulness. At that time, you turn down the volume of the mantra recording or even turn it off and follow with your own chant. Mantras such as *ram, hrim,* and *shrim* are perfect for vatas.

Pitta mantras should be soothing and cooling. *Om, aim, shrim,* and *sham* are great choices. They should be chanted during usual morning times (see "Training for the Pitta" in chapter VI) and also when emotions like anger increase. Whenever I have a short break between training my clients, I am always ready to step out for even five minutes next to the building, where under a tree I can chant my mantra and do a couple yoga postures to realign the energies.

Kapha mantras are *hum, aim,* and *om,* which all should be chanted or sung loudly. These mantras are warm and stimulating. Such mantras clear our cloudy perception of things. Congregational chanting and dancing is recommended, especially for those of kapha natures.

---

[21] Silent chanting means whispering and not "chanting in one's thoughts." Beginner stages and even intermediate stages of mantra-yoga require that we at least hear ourselves during chanting. This makes it is easier to keep the mind occupied with the mantra. Later, the mantra will become internalized by the practitioner.

Congregational chanting among like-minded individuals will definitely stir up energies you need to accomplish your worldly goals. Even as I am writing this sentence, our family is packing up for a yoga retreat in the mountains where there will be a lot of chanting and dancing, among other things. Everyone should plan their vacation keeping the principle of harmony in mind, so during such time we will actually recover from stress incurred during long months at work.

Herbal Supplementation Can Strengthen the Yoga-Mantra Practice

It is worth mentioning that certain herbs can improve perception, help open the energy channels, increase blood and oxygen flow to the brain, and therefore enhance one's mantra meditation experience. To this category belong calamus, tulsi, basil, bayberry, and sage. They can be taken with raw honey and warm water, which will magnify the herbal effect on your system.[22]

Yet other herbs can strengthen the intelligence and mind and build nerve tissue for better concentration and

---

[22] Ayurveda teaches that herbs work more efficiently when used in a synergistic way, or as a team of herbs with similar properties, as well as with carrier substances (water, honey, etc.).

absorption in the mantra chanting. They are shankhapushpi, brahmi, gotu kola, ashwagandha, haritaki, shatavari, bala, arjuna, lotus seeds, and shilajit. You can take them with warm raw (or lightly pasteurized) milk, raw sugar, raw honey, or clarified butter (ghee) to boost their energy.

The last category of meditation-enhancing herbs is for calming the mind. Usually our minds rush during chanting and we have two tracks running, one for chanting and another one for whatever the mind brings. When you slow the mind down, you will be able to hear the sound vibration more distinctly. These herbs are jatamansi, valerian, nutmeg, kava kava, lady's slipper, and skullcap. You can take these herbs along with aloe gel or ghee.

Optimum Amount of Tension in the Systems (OATS)

Our body-mind system is in constant flux, and even though it sometimes may seem still (e.g., when we do not move or we sleep), it is always running at different levels. Perfect stillness is not plausible at the physical or subtle level due to the nature of forces engaged, nor is erratic movement possible long term since it causes quick exhaustion of the forces. Optimum flow of Prana is the one that prolongs the functioning of its constituent parts.

The ancient knowledge of Ayurveda lists various physiological systems in the body, which are called *shrotamsi* in Sanskrit. The 14 *shrotamsi* more or less correspond to the systems of Western medicine and are like irrigation channels, providing nutrients necessary for us to thrive and carrying away toxins we do not need. They are the respiratory system, digestive system, water-metabolism system, sweating system, excretory system, urinary system, lymphatic system, circulatory system, muscular system, adipose system (fat), skeletal system, nervous system, reproductive system, and mental system. As mentioned in chapter IV, in "The Five Vayus Related to Physical Tissues and Channels," each phase and type of breathing will have an effect on certain physiological channels and the mental channel. Furthermore, each marma manipulation will have an effect on certain physiological channels as well. Finally, mantra pronunciation will affect the channels, especially the mental system and higher chakras.

The proper practice of combative arts according to our mental and physical constitution entails the usage of body-mind specific nutrition, training, breathing techniques, marma manipulation, and hearing of mantra. Only by such practice of martial arts can we restore, raise, and preserve the optimum amount of tension of the five types of Chi and the three doshas within each system so that everything flows in harmony. Each martial artist will do the best service to himself/herself if they eat their daily OATS. As in the words of sage Lao Tsu,

Know the strength of man,
but keep a woman's care!
Be the stream of the universe!
Being the stream of the universe,
ever true and unswerving,
become as a little child once more.

Know the white,
but keep the black!
Be an example to the world!
Being an example to the world,
ever true and unwavering,
return to the infinite.

Know honor,
yet keep humility.
Be the valley of the universe!
Being the valley of the universe,
ever true and resourceful,
return to the state of the uncarved block. (28)

Chapter VI

Warrior Daily Planner

General Strategy for Harmonious Martial Arts Training

To experience an elevated mental state during one's martial arts training and achieve great results afterward, one needs to look at one's mental and physical constitution to determine which times will generally be best for such practice. For example, a vata will feel more grounded, confident, and strong training during pitta and kapha hours of the day, which are between 6 a.m. and 2 p.m. That is very important in the realm of martial arts. Anything earlier or later should be used for yoga/meditation or, in other words, for stabilization of Prana. A junction between kapha and pitta times (9 a.m. to 10 a.m.) works as well.

A pitta training at pitta and vata times, which are between 10 a.m. and 6 p.m., will feel more aggressive, powerful, and fast as well, which are great assets to most warriors. A junction time between pitta and vata works too (2 p.m. to 3 p.m.). Anything earlier or later will be a trade-off for less speed, more lethargy, etc. Those times should be used for yoga/meditation and harmonizing of Prana.

A kapha training at pitta and vata times listed above (but finishing a little earlier) will enhance his/her speed, reflexes, and aggressiveness. Since the kapha tends to already be strong and grounded, they will benefit from enhancing the qualities they may not possess to a high degree. A junction time between vata and pitta times works well (2 p.m. to 3 p.m.), but anything earlier or later will shift the kapha into much slower gears. Therefore, yoga/meditation is recommended at that time.

All of the guidelines given below aim at avoiding intense physical training during times of either mental slowness or increased body-type-like qualities that may throw us out of the circle of harmony. Mental slowness manifests during morning and evening kapha times (6 a.m. to 10 a.m. and 6 p.m. to 10 p.m.). Between 5 p.m. and midnight, when the mode of ignorance is dominant, the intelligence tends to be more easily bewildered. The guidelines assume that qualities of vata and pitta are more conducive to combative training than kapha qualities and that training itself is vigorous.

An additional consideration for choosing one's training time is the type of martial arts training to be done (speed training, reflex training, strength training, functional sparring). Someone who is a vata and who is working on speed might as well try the vata time period, which they should normally avoid. He/she might set a record that day and be in need of more energy balancing afterward! However, the same type of warrior who is supposed to have a strength workout will be better off choosing a pitta or even kapha time range. Or someone of a pitta constitution who is working on semi-contact tae kwon do type of sparring might also consider the vata time period, since aggressiveness and strength will take second place to speed and reaction time for that particular workout.

Training for the Vata

As you recall from chapter I, the abundant elements in the vata body type are air and ether, but there is an inherent lack of fire, water, and earth. You must carefully control your strengths (air, ether) and nourish your weaknesses (fire, water, earth). Having a vata physical body and mental disposition gives you the lightning speed advantage both in body and mind over other types and predisposes you to burning yourself out quickly. You may have great cardiovascular endurance but it is hard for you to back it up with strength. Trying to work on too many things at once can be a challenge for you, as can being consistent with whatever task you undertake. If you desire to feel the right kind of power every time you train, you must allow ample time for the recovery phase. Ample time in the recovery phase does not mean sitting idly but incorporating vata-balancing exercises and routines that you do on off days. Those build total strength and add grounding to your mental battlefield.

Vata-Harmonizing Martial Arts Practice Worked into a Daily Routine [23]

6 a.m. to 7 a.m. This is the ideal wake-up time for a vata warrior. It is very important to begin their day by rising promptly after awakening to take a warm, even hot, shower (especially in the wintertime). Scraping the tongue of toxins accumulated overnight and drinking two cups of warm lemon water will ignite their digestion gradually. Cleansing the nasal passages via the neti pot will ensure that their breathing and thinking during stretching practice will be maximized. Alternate-nostril breathing is recommended especially if feeling either inertia (excess ether) or agitation (excess air). Placing vata-controlling oils on the body, such as high-quality sesame oil, is recommended.

7 a.m. to 8 a.m. Powerful yoga postures to be implemented include, for the less flexible fighters, runner's lunge, wall

---

[23]Times and some routine activities adapted from Tiwari, 187–89.

push, power-chair, triangle, warrior I, boat pose, bridge pose, child's pose, staff pose, head-to-knee pose, hero, and alligator twists. For the more flexible fighters, the following can be added: extended side angle pose, warrior III, intense back extension pose, upward single leg forward bend, full shoulder stand, unsupported cobra, reclining hero pose, open legs forward bend. For very flexible fighters, additional poses are introduced such as revolving triangle, headstand, plow pose, and revolving head-to-knee pose.

The stretching practice should take at least 45 minutes and be followed by more specific breathing techniques such as the right-nostril breathing, which increases vital fires in the body.

The morning time before breakfast is a great time to focus on technique-oriented movements. After doing yoga, the martial artist can do their forms, hone on single techniques, do a few sets of energy-stabilizing stances or techniques such as the horse rider stance, simple kicks, and punches. The session should leave one feeling grounded and powered up.

8 a.m. to 9 a.m. A medium-sized breakfast will consist of vata-friendly foods (see the charts in chapter III). Vatas have a tendency to rush out of home, skipping breakfast all together, but that may unbalance them later in the morning. In general, they do not do well without breakfast, as they run out of energy quickly. The vata warrior will remember to focus on the task at hand when eating, while reducing talking, checking the phone, listening to news, etc. It is not only what is eaten but how it is eaten. The mindset during a meal will affect assimilation of nutrients and determine if any subtle toxins will form in the subtle counterpart of his/her personality. The less toxins one accumulates in the subtle realm of mind and intelligence, the swifter one's mind will operate during training and daily activities.

9 a.m. to 2 p.m. This is a good time to perform work-related activities that culminate in a rich lunch composed of vata-friendly foods. If preparing for some event, whether a fight or show in the coming months, the vata will perform cardiovascular activities in the morning hours after eating a hearty breakfast (at least one and a half to two hours after breakfast). Assuming they have done some yoga already, a 30-minute run would suffice. The run could reflect some of the specifics they are working on, such as intervals of running, rope skipping, and shadow fighting.

The lunch should be eaten in a peaceful atmosphere, chewed slowly, and enjoyed. If no workout was performed in the morning (except for yoga stretches), then early lunch (around 11 a.m.) is preferable. If a workout was done after a good breakfast, then lunch can be eaten at noon or a little later. Since this is a time of increased fire in the atmosphere, a wise vata will try to perform most of the important tasks of the day.

A martial arts event in the late morning or at around noon will be compatible with the vata constitution as long as a hearty breakfast was consumed earlier. A warrior of vata constitution could get away with eating a light lunch one and a half to two hours before the match.

The schedule can be adjusted in the following way: Performing morning yoga stretches and meditations but skipping the technical workout or cardio is a smart move, as is eating a more solid breakfast (if fighting before lunch). Ideally the competition event should happen before lunch when the warrior feels light yet fired up and his/her mind is sharp. Wise warriors do not exert themselves when hungry or thirsty.

A slower-pace, event-specific warm-up is good to avoid injury, as vatas possess great speed. For example, if a person is about to compete in semi-contact kumite (tae kwon do or kung-fu style) and strikes with full speed on a cold engine, some parts may tear (tendons, muscles).

2 p.m. to 5 p.m. This time of the day is used for rejuvenation of life force and grounding. Vatas require more recovery time, as they have more delicate frameworks and edgy minds. Recommended activities include listening to pleasant sounds (nature or music), meditating, remaining in quietude for some time, taking a nap, and doing gentle yoga stretches. If more work remains to be done that day, a cup of vata-friendly tea would not be bad.

5 p.m. to 7 p.m. One does the remaining work of the day. The focus is on reflecting about today and planning ahead. An early supper composed of vata-recommended foods could be at 6 p.m. with friends and family.

7 p.m. to 10 p.m. Walking in the park or garden, watching tropical fish in a tank, or doing some other relaxing activity is good for vatas at this time. Breathing exercises meant to quiet the mind are to be performed at this time as well. Many vatas do well with aromas of essential oils or incense, which, when diffused in the room, can help adopt a certain mood.

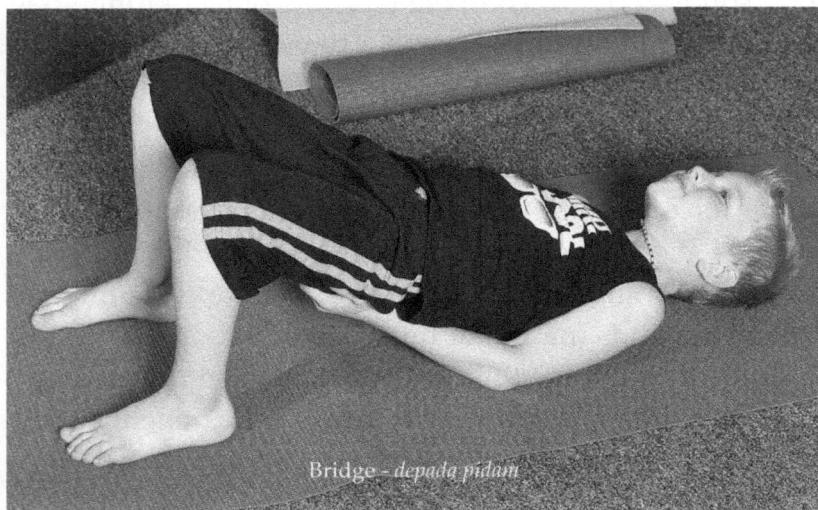

Bridge – *depada pidam*

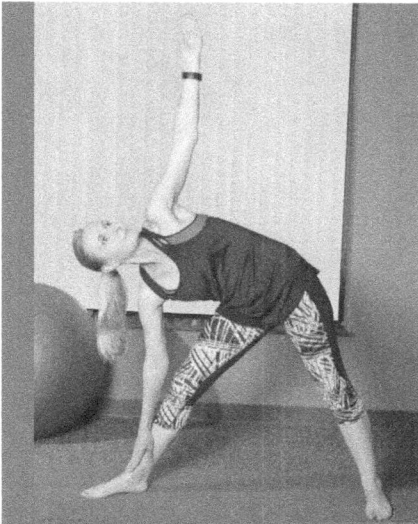

Triangle - *trikonasana*

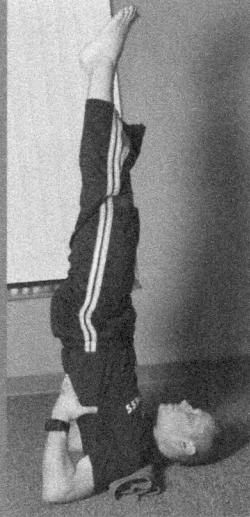

Shoulder Stand
- *sarvangasana III*

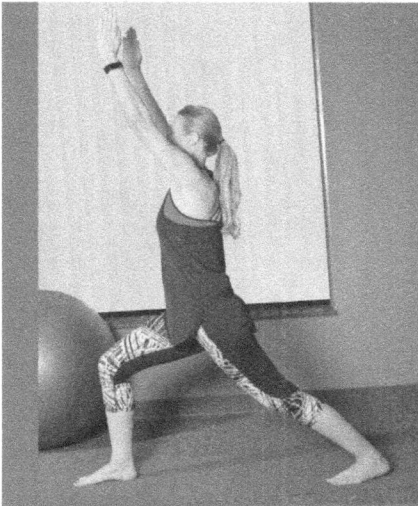

Warrior I - *virabhadrasana I*

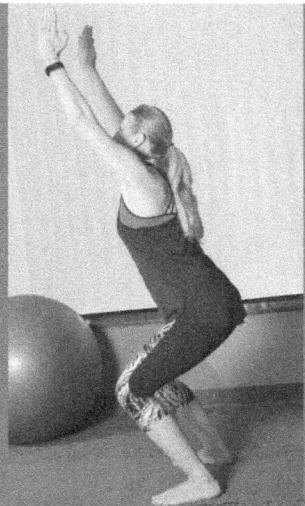

Power chair - *utkatasana*

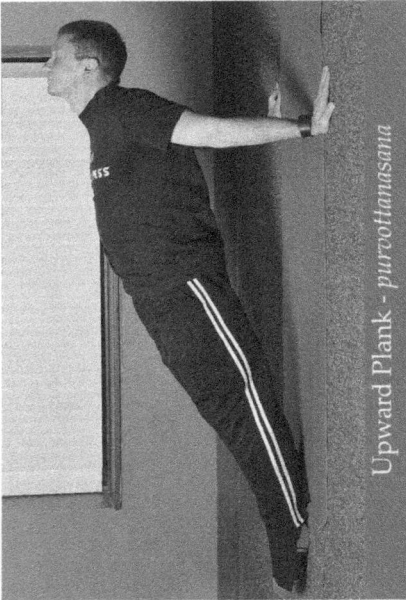

Upward Plank - *purvottanasana*

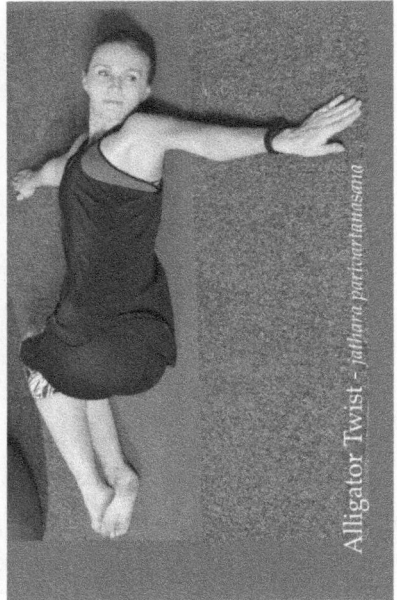

Alligator Twist - *jathara parivartanasana*

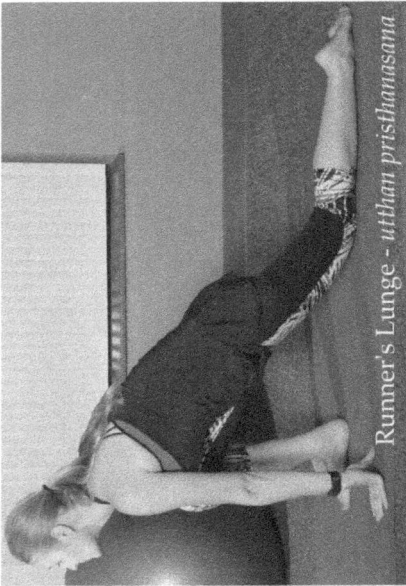

Runner's Lunge - *utthan pristhanasana*

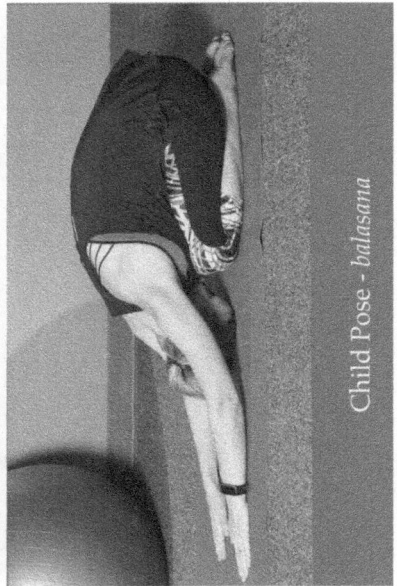

Child Pose - *balasana*

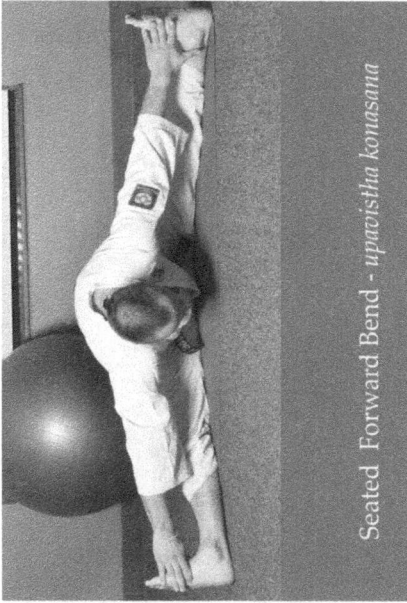

Seated Forward Bend - *upavistha konasana*

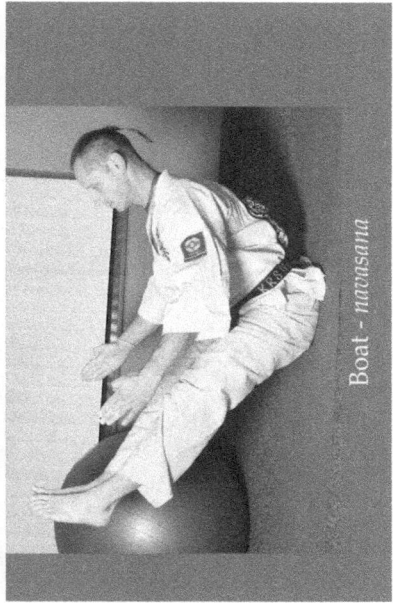

Boat - *navasana*

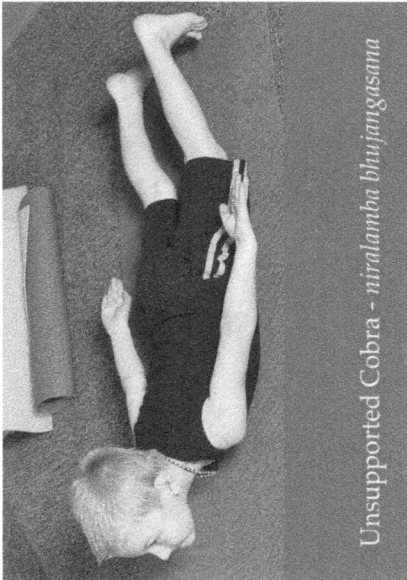

Unsupported Cobra - *niralamba bhujangasana*

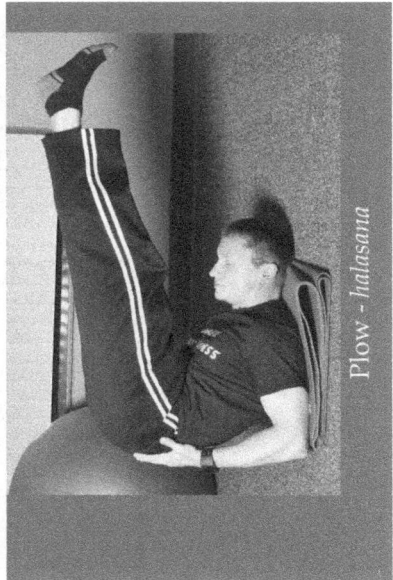

Plow - *halasana*

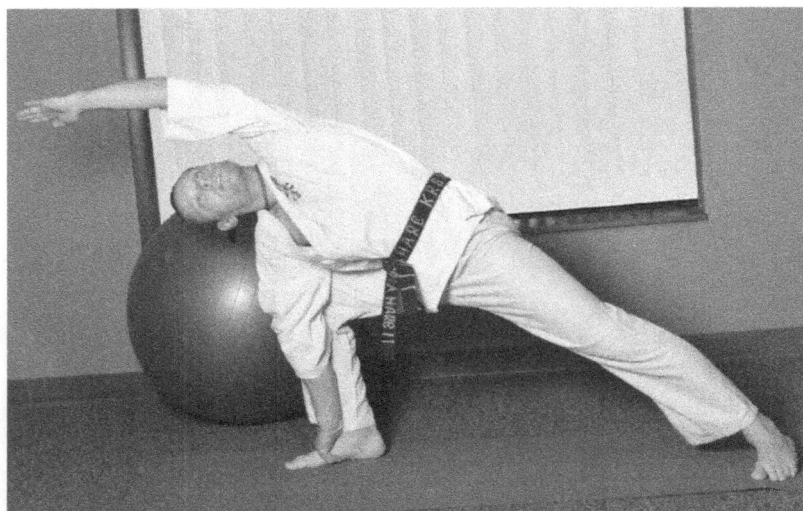

Extended Side Angle - *parsvakonasana*

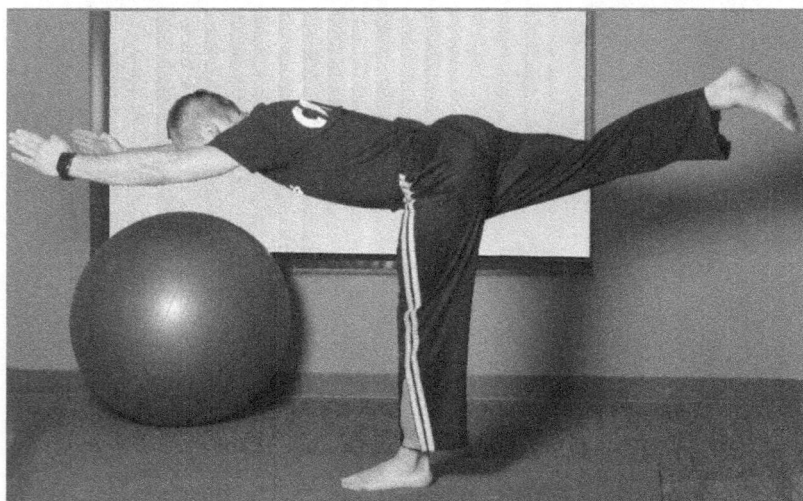

Warrior III - *virabhadrasana III*

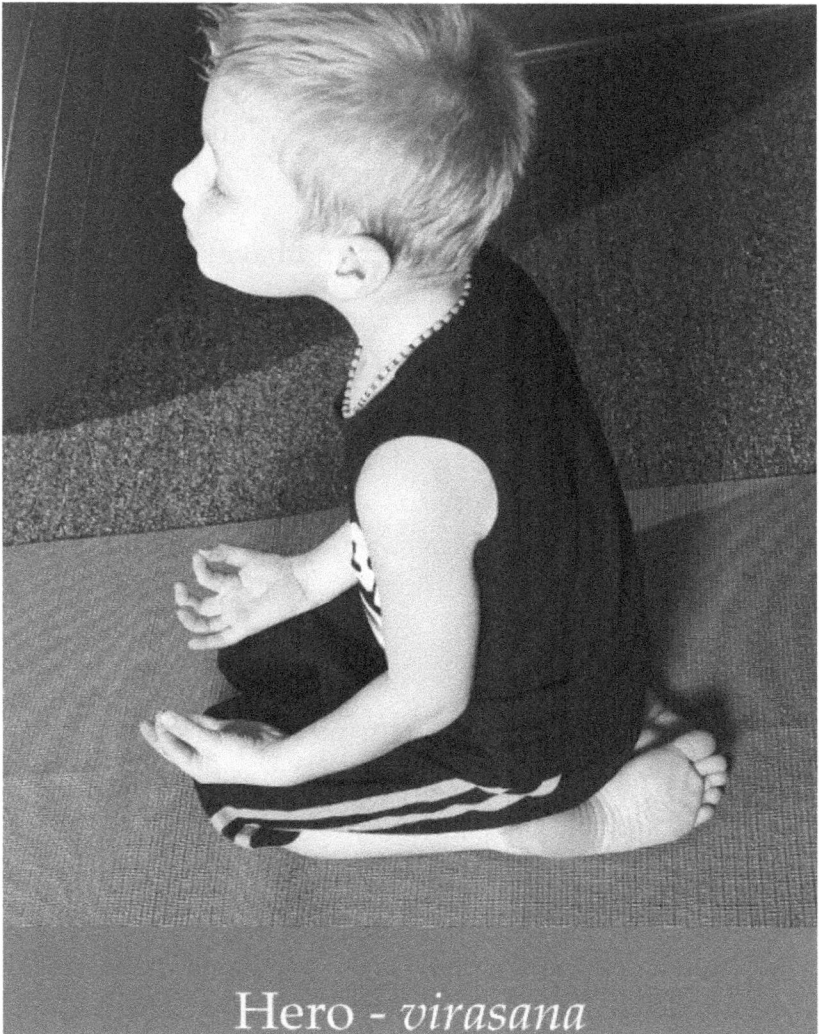

Hero - *virasana*

Training for the Pitta

In the Ayurvedic view, the pitta warrior has an abundance of fire and water but naturally lacks air, ether, and earth. You must restrain your fire and water while augmenting the weaknesses (air, ether, earth). If you are a pitta, you naturally carry with you a great amount of striking power. You are also fast and have decent muscle endurance and cardiovascular fitness. In order for you to feel the right kind of power when training, you must avoid overheating your engine. It is essential for you to perform your workouts at times when there is not much heat in the atmosphere. It is also crucial that you perform your pitta-balancing exercises and routines before your workout session. Those increase coolness of mind and relax the body to enhance efficiency of power usage.

Pitta-Harmonizing Martial Arts Practice
Worked into a Daily Routine

5:30 a.m. to 6:30 a.m. A pitta warrior begins his/her day by rising promptly after awakening to take a cool shower. Scraping the tongue of toxins accumulated overnight and drinking one to two cups of cool lemon water will ignite their digestion gradually. Cleansing the nasal passages via the neti pot will ensure that their breathing and thinking during stretching practice will be maximized. Placing fire-reducing oils on the body, such as virgin unrefined coconut oil, is recommended.

6:30 a.m. to 8 a.m. Begin by performing the alternate-nostril breathing, which improves communication between the right and left brain hemispheres. Powerful yoga postures to be implemented include, for the less flexible fighters, cat stretch, downward dog, runner's lunge, standing spinal twist, child's pose, one-legged stretch lying down, head-to-knee pose, alligator twist, corpse pose. For the more flexible fighters, the following can be added: standing sun god, spread legs forward bend, half shoulder stand, revolved head-to-knee pose, cobra stretch, open leg forward bend. For very flexible fighters, additional poses are introduced such as handstand, full shoulder stand, reclining hero pose, and full forward bend. The stretching practice should take at least 20 minutes. If excessive energy or aggression is perceived, then left-nostril breathing is recommended.

If preparing for some event, whether a fight or show in the coming months, the pitta warrior will do some cardiovascular training in the morning hours before eating a solid breakfast. He/she will remember not to overdo it and deplete themselves of energy too early in the day. Assuming they have done some yoga already, a 30-minute run is more than sufficient. The run should be pleasant, and sweating should be moderate. The run could reflect some of the specifics they are working on, such as intervals of running and rope skipping, or running and shadow fighting.

The morning time before breakfast is also a great time to focus on technique-oriented movements. After doing yoga, the martial artist can do their forms, hone on single techniques, or do a few hundred of the same punch, block, or kick. They must remember not to overexert themselves. The session should leave one feeling satisfied with their work and their start to the day.

8 a.m. to 9 a.m. A medium-sized breakfast will consist of pitta-friendly foods (see the charts in chapter III). Pittas do not do well without breakfast, as the hunger pangs may get too intense and throw off their focus. The pitta warrior will remember to think about pleasant and relaxing things, events, and persons when eating. It is not only what is eaten but how it is eaten. The mindset during a meal will affect assimilation of nutrients and determine if any subtle toxins will form in the subtle counterpart of his/her personality. The less toxins one accumulates in the subtle realm of mind and intelligence, the clearer one's mind will operate during training and daily activities.

9 a.m. to 1 p.m. This is a good time to perform work-related activities that culminate in a hearty lunch of pitta-friendly foods. Since this is a time of increased fire in the atmosphere, a smart pitta warrior will try to do even-tempered work and stay clear of stressful situations, as they might easily throw him/her off-balance. Emphasis on care for others and using one's strong will to control anger and ambition will ensure a successful day.

A martial arts event in the late morning or at around noon will give the pitta an added power advantage due to the prevalence of fire and water elements in the atmosphere. The fire element is the most important element in martial arts such as karate and kickboxing. Other types of martial arts (tai chi, aikido, jujitsu) may align more with earth, water, ether, and air, which would give subtle functional advantages at different times of the day to their practitioners.

The schedule can be adjusted in the following way: Performing morning yoga stretches and meditations but skipping the technical workout or cardio is a smart move, as is eating a more solid breakfast. Ideally the competition should happen even before lunch when the warrior feels light yet fired up and his/her mind is sharp. Wise warriors do not exert themselves when hungry or thirsty.

A medium-intensity, event-specific warm-up is good to do to avoid injury due to the great anaerobic power pittas possess. For example, if a person is about to compete in full-contact kumite (karate style) and launches that power with a still cold engine, some parts (tendons, ligaments, muscles) may snap.

1 p.m. to 6 p.m. This time can be devoted to work-related activities, with emphasis on communicating with others (if aspects of a job call for it), and assessing the day (in terms of what was productive or unproductive). He/she checks off their list of duties for the day. Somewhere in that time range it is good to take a half-hour break if needed for tea or a medium-sized protein snack (if hunger levels are noticeably high due to physical exertion earlier).

6 p.m. to 7 p.m. This is for suppertime with good company. That means a sensible warrior does not overeat. The physical body will get the best rest if it is not overloaded with a lot of dense foods at this time. Consulting a pitta-constitution food chart is a great way to go. Depending on how much the warrior worked out earlier and depending on their hunger level, the meal quantity should be adjusted. Now is a good time to take a walk and do activities that are calming. A result-oriented warrior will also plan for tomorrow but will not be obsessed with tomorrow.

Evening time is by no means a good time for training the body hard, competing, or anything of that sort. The fire element is prevalent in the atmosphere as is the quality of dullness (*tamas*, or "ignorance"), which will hamper any practice and affect the rest period for the body-mind system. Whether one seemingly succeeds or not in the evening practice is not the point. The important thing is that martial arts practice (other than light forms of it like tai chi or breathing exercises) in the evening is bound to aggravate the fire elements, which are already strongly present in the warrior, resulting in or contributing to loss of harmony.

7 p.m. to 9 p.m. A pitta works smart when he/she reduces activities early in the evening. The sooner and more one reduces their daily activities as the sun comes down, the better rest their body-mind system will get. The brain gets most of its rest between 10 p.m. and midnight. So one should relax and read something they like that does not overly excite them.

9 p.m. to 10 p.m. This is a good time for a short session of calming yoga poses, incense (e.g., sandalwood), breathing exercises, and meditation. One should retire shortly after

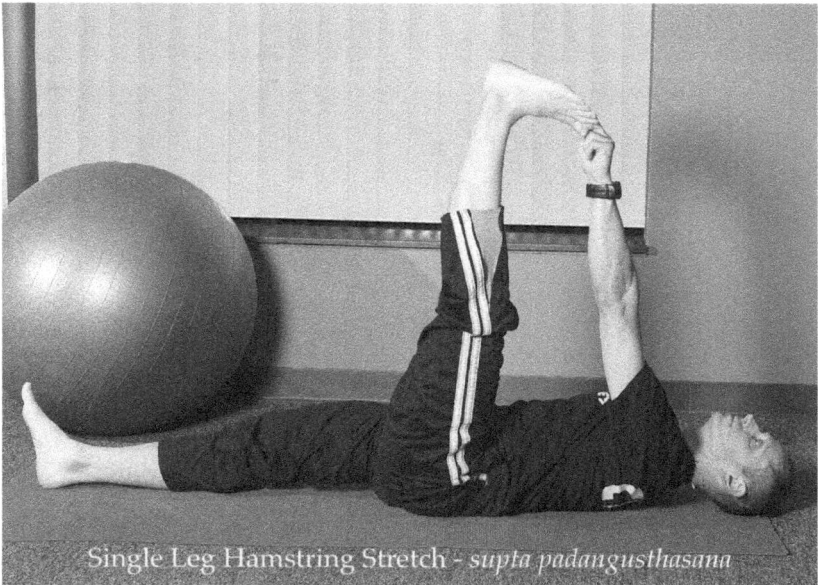

Single Leg Hamstring Stretch - *supta padangusthasana*

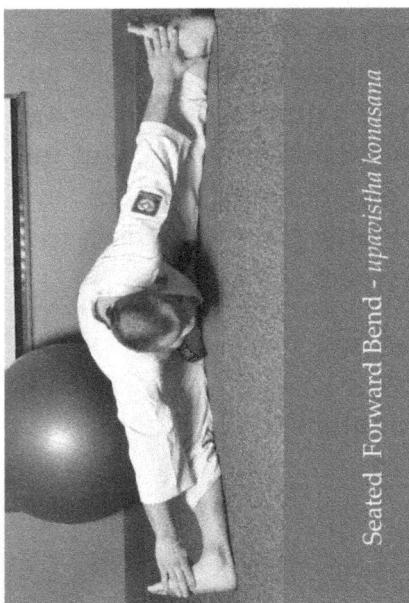

Seated Forward Bend - *upavistha konasana*

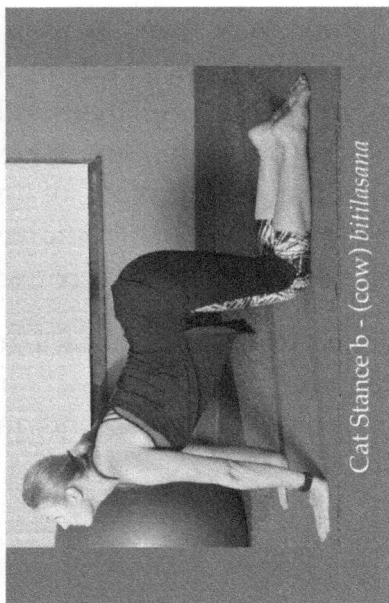

Cat Stance b - (cow) *bitilasana*

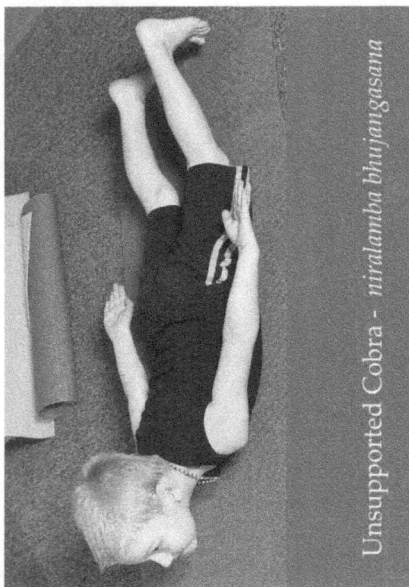

Unsupported Cobra - *niralamba bhujangasana*

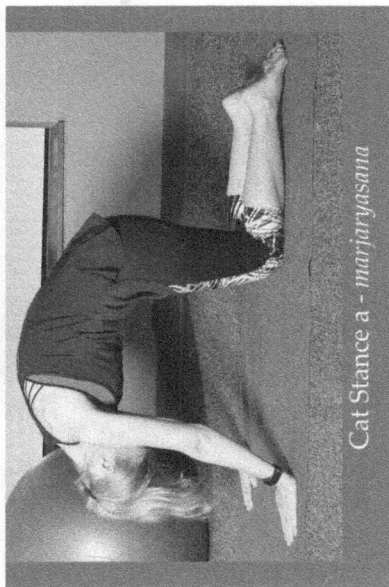

Cat Stance a - *marjaryasana*

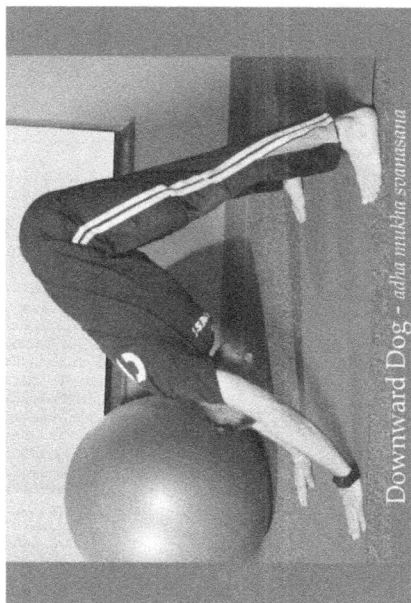

Downward Dog - *adha mukha svanasana*

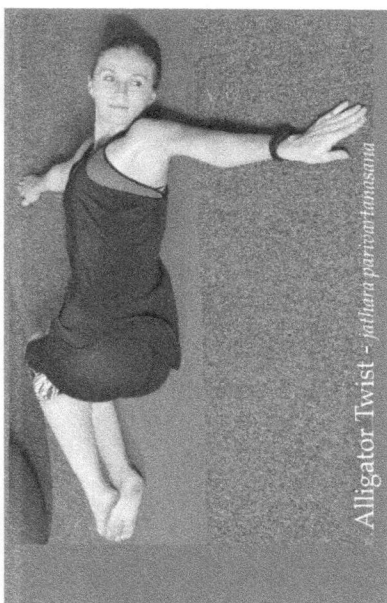

Alligator Twist - *jathara parivartanasana*

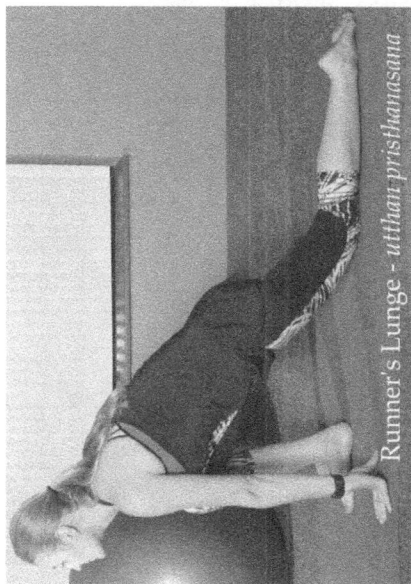

Runner's Lunge - *utthan pristhanasana*

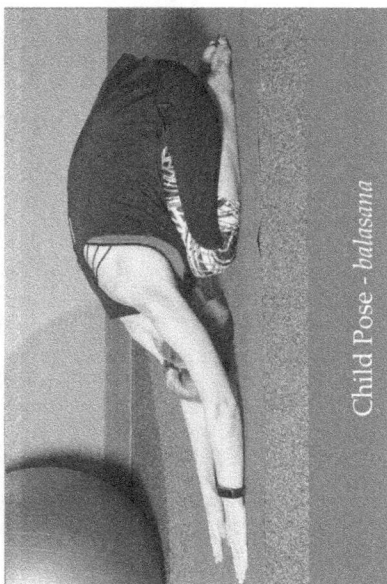

Child Pose - *balasana*

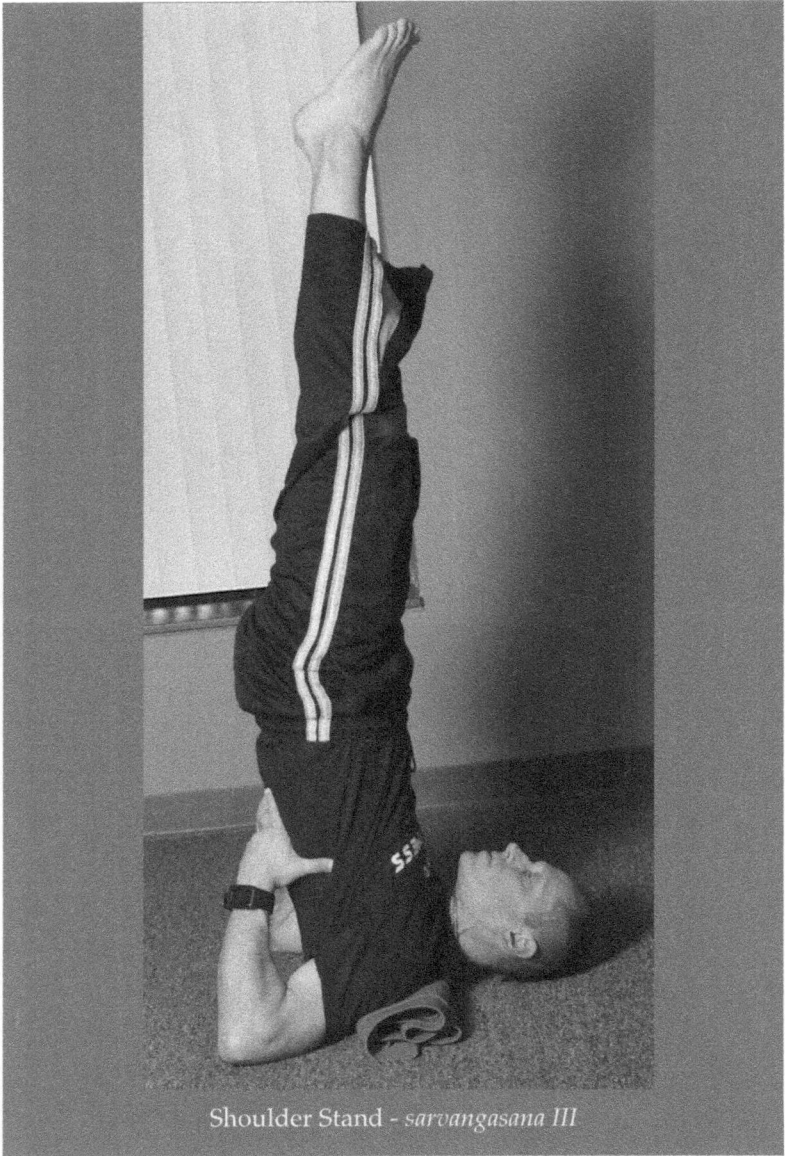

Shoulder Stand - *sarvangasana III*

Training for the Kapha

According to Ayurveda, a kapha warrior naturally possesses water and earth elements but lacks air, ether, and fire. Therefore, he/she should aim at increasing air, ether, fire and controlling the water and earth. Having a kapha body certainly gives you an advantage of total strength as well as life force endurance. The weakness that you may or may not be aware of is lesser speed and, therefore, power that is an essential factor in many of the martial arts. It may also be hard for you to get started on a new training routine or just get enough workouts in per week. You can certainly benefit from buddy training or simply someone who will remind and motivate you or literally drag you to the dojo. It is of utmost importance that kaphas perform invigorating kapha-balancing exercises that ignite their fire to last through the workout. Without enhancing the fire, you will not be able to use the great strength that you possess in the martial arts.

Kapha-Harmonizing Martial Arts Practice Worked into a Daily Routine

4:30 a.m. to 5:30 a.m. This is the ideal wake-up time for a kapha warrior. It is very important to begin his/her day by rising promptly after awakening to take a warm shower. Scraping the tongue of toxins accumulated overnight and drinking one cup of warm lemon water will ignite their digestion gradually. Cleansing the nasal passages via the neti pot will ensure that their breathing and thinking during stretching practice will be maximized. Placing fire-enhancing oils on the body, such as high-quality mustard oil, is recommended.

5:30 a.m. to 8 a.m. Begin by performing the alternate-nostril breathing to reduce lethargy or intertia. Powerful yoga postures to be implemented include, for the less flexible fighters, standing sun god, downward dog, warrior I, warrior II, half shoulder stand, unsupported cobra variations, boat pose, bridge pose, and alligator twists. For the more flexible fighters, the following can be added: runner's lunge, triangle pose, revolving triangle pose, half-moon pose, warrior III, chest opening exercise by the wall, upward leg forward bend, intense back extension pose, and headstand. For very flexible fighters, additional poses are introduced such as handstand, bow pose, upward bow pose, side plank pose, single-legged supine hamstring stretch, and revolved head-to-knee pose.

The stretching practice should take at least 30 minutes and be followed by more specific breathing techniques such as right-nostril breathing, which increases vital fires in the body.

If preparing for some event, whether a fight or show in the coming months, the kapha will do intense cardiovascular activities in the morning hours before eating a very light breakfast. Pushing hard during the cardio sessions will set their energy right for most of the day. Assuming they have done some yoga already, a 45-minute run would suffice. The run could reflect some of the specifics they are working on, such as intervals of running and rope skipping, shadow fighting, and even pushing tires, pulling sleds, and throwing heavy medicine balls.

The morning time before breakfast is also a great time to focus on technique-oriented movements. After doing yoga, the martial artist can do their forms, hone on single techniques, and do a few hundred of the same punch, block, or kick. The session should leave one feeling fired up and ready to seize the day.

8 a.m. to 9 a.m. A small-sized breakfast will consist of kapha-friendly foods (see the charts in chapter III). It is also advised that kapha skip breakfast entirely or just drink a glass of green juice consisting of kapha-friendly foods, which will stir up their latent energies. Feeling a little hunger and waiting till lunch is not a bad proposal for a kapha. It should be reiterated that the mindset during a meal will affect assimilation of nutrients and determine if any subtle toxins will form in the subtle spirit counterpart of his/her personality. The less toxins one accumulates in the subtle realm of mind and intelligence, the clearer one's mind will operate during training and daily activities.

9 a.m. to 2 p.m. This is a good time to perform work-related activities that culminate in a hearty lunch of kapha-friendly foods. If there is a martial arts event in the late morning or at around noon that the warrior participates in, then the schedule can be adjusted in the following way: Performing morning yoga stretches and meditations but skipping the technical workout along with breakfast is a smart move for the Kapha warrior. Ideally the competition event should happen before lunch when the warrior feels light yet fired up and his/her mind is sharp.

Kaphas will need a more-intense event-specific warm-up before because their fire element is a minor factor. They need to spend more time igniting it. For example, performing punches and kicks with 70 to 80 percent power for 10 to 15 minutes, with short breaks in between sets, would be all right. Such a warm-up might feel like a workout to a vata or pitta, but it will be perfect for a kapha before they go all out.

2 p.m. to 7 p.m. Since the ether and air elements are prevalent in the atmosphere at this time, kaphas should use this time to perform the hardest tasks of their jobs. This will give them the extra wind they do not have in the morning or evening hours. It is also a good idea to drink some spicy tea to accelerate the surge of energy. An appropriate time to do that is 4 p.m. to 4:30 p.m.

Because the fire element is still present but slowly

decreasing after 2 p.m. and the air and ether elements are rising in influence, a time range between 2 p.m. and 4 p.m. would be a very good time for kaphas to compete. A shorter and less-intense warm-up might suffice. At that time, the air, ether, and fire elements are completing kapha's weaker spots. In contrast, when kaphas compete in the morning, they may still lack the functional principle of mobility, and when they compete in the late afternoon, although the light energy of air and ether will still be present, the earth and water elements and the mode of ignorance will already be building up. For a kapha, who already has a dominance of water and earth, that might prove quite disarming.

7 p.m. to 8 p.m. This is time for a light dinner with friends and family.

8 p.m. to 10 p.m. Kaphas should perform somewhat intense kapha-specific yoga poses or even a light group martial arts practice. Because kaphas require the fire element to feel harmonized, a more intense practice in the evening will not overstimulate or tire them to the same degree as it would a vata or pitta. It must be remembered, though, that dinner time and quantity should be adjusted —such as by eating earlier or by cutting portions in half— to allow two hours for at least the first stage of digestion to occur. The yoga practice, workout, or martial arts practice should not last past 10 p.m.

10 p.m. to 11 p.m. This is a good time to relax and perform some evening meditation. One should go to sleep shortly after.

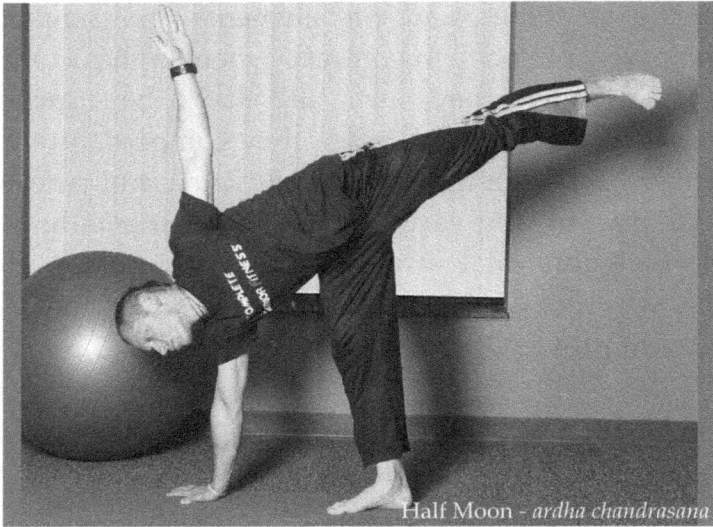

Half Moon - *ardha chandrasana*

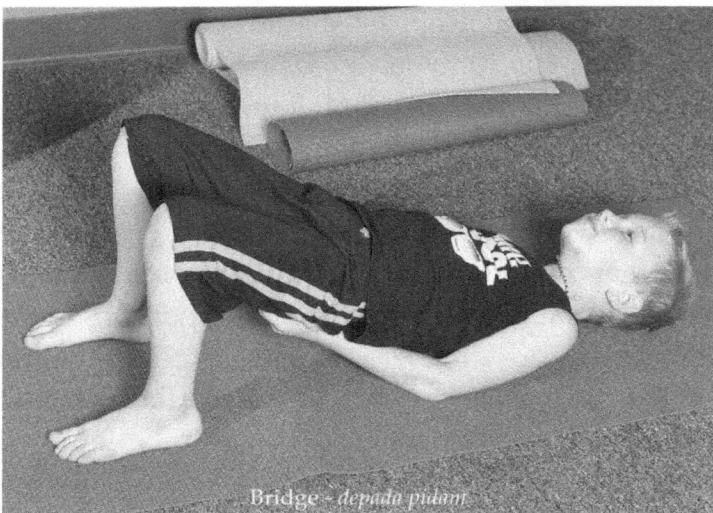

Bridge - *depada pidam*

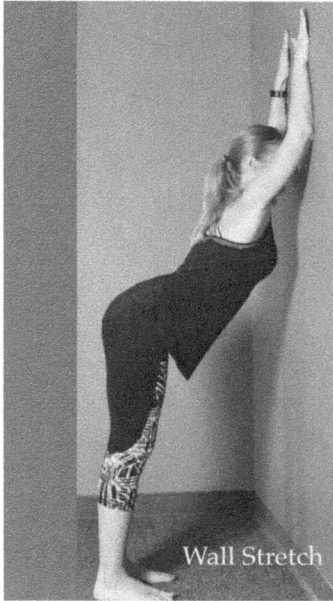

Wall Stretch

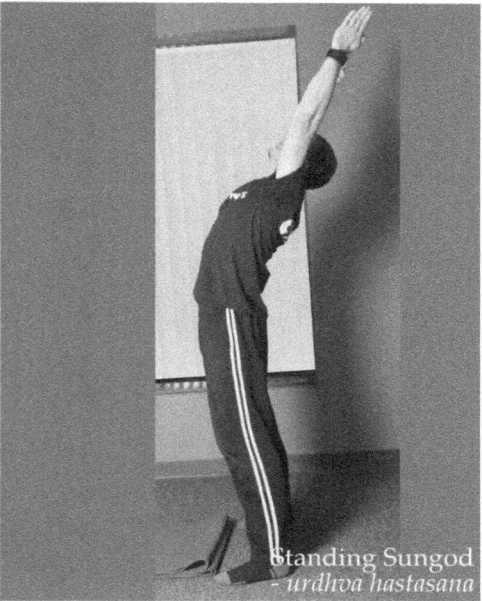

Standing Sungod
- *urdhva hastasana*

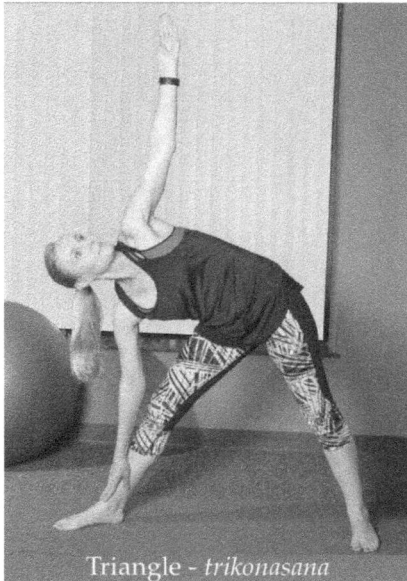

Triangle - *trikonasana*

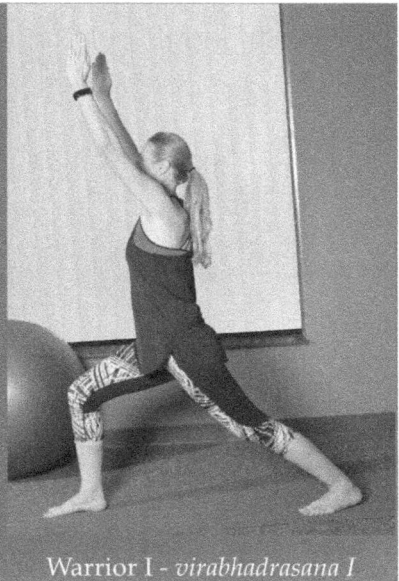

Warrior I - *virabhadrasana I*

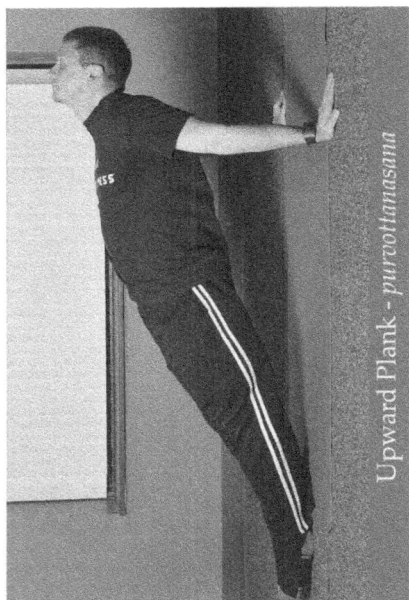

Upward Plank - *purvottanasana*

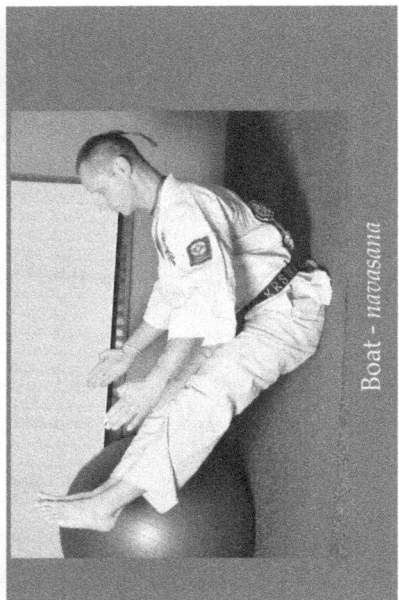

Boat - *navasana*

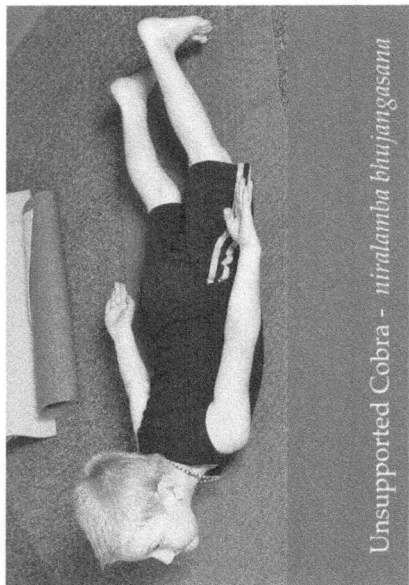

Unsupported Cobra - *niralamba bhujangasana*

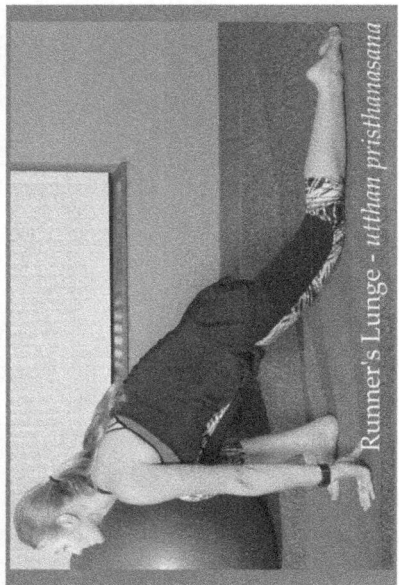

Runner's Lunge - *utthan pristhanasana*

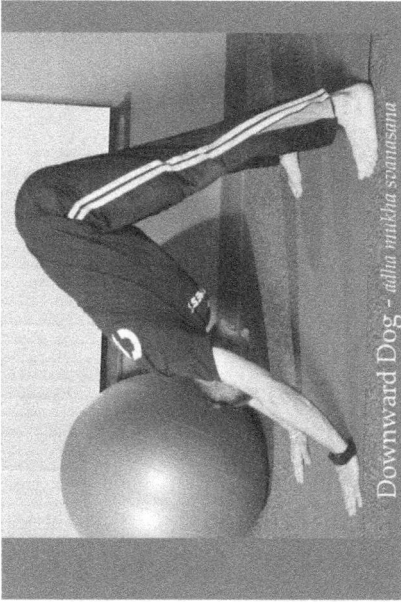

Downward Dog - *adha mukha svanasana*

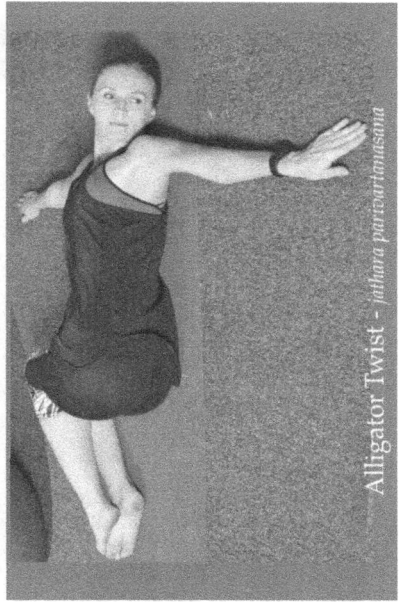

Alligator Twist - *jathara parivartanasana*

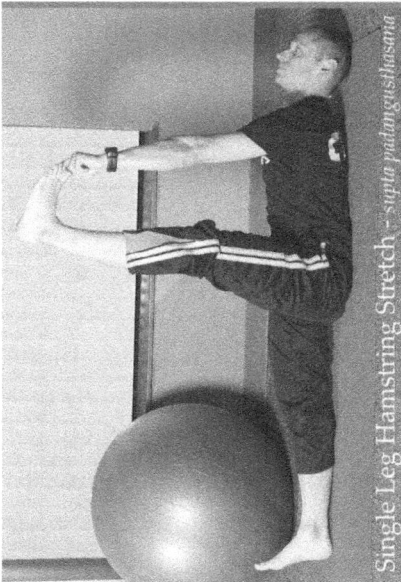

Single Leg Hamstring Stretch - *supta padangusthasana*

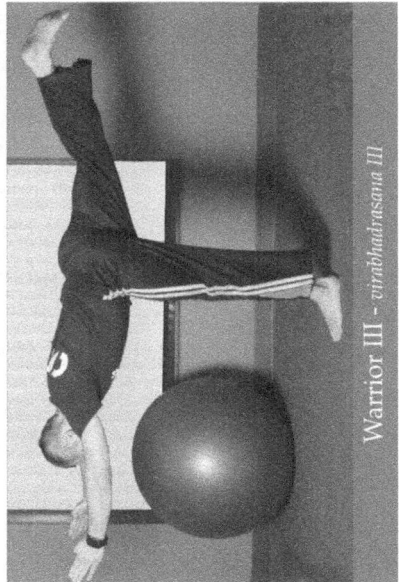

Warrior III - *virabhadrasana III*

Mixed Types

If you are a pure vata, pitta, or kapha, then you are, we can say, lucky. You will have less factors, such as seasonal, dietary, and other changes, that interfere with your innate balance. Most of us will have two dominant natures, one of them usually somewhat stronger than the other.

Training for Vata-Pittas

If you are primarily a fairly even combination of vata and pitta, then you must determine if the differences are aligned more physically (bone and muscle structure) or subtly (actions of mind and intellect).

If you are physically mostly a vata but your thinking and emotional patterns are that of a pPitta, then your nutrition should fulfill more the pitta nature, whereas your yoga practice should focus on harmonizing the vata. Similarly, those of a pitta body type but vata nature will eat more like vatas but do yoga according to pitta guidelines.

With the change of seasons from summer to fall, one who is of dual nature will have to switch his/her focus from harmonizing pitta (fire) to harmonizing vata (air).

As a VP, you will usually have a poorer level of circulation and like heat but have a limited ability to endure it. You may have a very strong appetite, but your digestive acid may not be strong enough to handle a large meal. At the emotional level, when you are exposed to stress, you may oscillate between bouts of anger and anxiety. You are both light and intense, which is a great asset to a martial artist, and to any athlete for that matter. The best way to harmonize your unique body type at the physical level is the adding of earth and water elements via the intake of proper foods and right exercise routines, while the best way to harmonize at the emotional level is the intake of grounding images (mantra meditation). Breathing techniques that focus on increasing stability include left-nostril breathing and Vyana and Samana Vayu techniques.

6 a.m. to 7 a.m. This is the ideal wake-up time for a VP warrior. It is very important to begin his/her day by rising promptly after awakening to take a warm to cool shower depending on the season. Scraping the tongue of toxins accumulated overnight and drinking one to two cups of warm lemon water will ignite their digestion gradually. Cleansing the nasal passages via the neti pot will ensure that their breathing and thinking during stretching practice will be maximized. Alternate-nostril breathing is recommended at this point. Placing good oils on the body, such as high-quality sesame oil or coconut oil, is recommended.

7 a.m. to 8 a.m. Powerful yoga postures to be implemented include a combination of stretches for vatas and pittas.

Please refer back to those two sections. The stretching practice should take at least 45 minutes and be followed by more specific breathing techniques such as the right-nostril breathing, which increases vital fires in the body. One can consult the section on breathing for the five types of Chi to pick the breathing sequence that suits your type and current needs. For example, if one is struggling with anxiety before an important event that's coming up, it would be wise to enhance Udana Vayu and Apana Vayu, since they are responsible for the ability to express oneself in the world as well as the ability to neutralize negative thinking patterns born of constantly incoming mental images.

The morning time before breakfast is a great time to focus on technique-oriented movements. After doing yoga, the martial artist should do their forms, hone on single techniques, or do a few sets of energy-stabilizing stances or techniques such as the horse rider stance, simple kicks, and punches. The session should leave one feeling grounded and powered-up.

8 a.m. to 9 a.m. A medium-sized breakfast will consist of vata-friendly foods. If one has a tendency to rush out of home skipping breakfast, that may unbalance them later in the morning. One should be mindful to focus on the task at hand when eating, while reducing talking, checking the phone, listening to news, etc. It is not only what is eaten but how it is eaten. The mindset during a meal will affect assimilation of nutrients and determine if any subtle toxins will form in the subtle spirit counterpart of his/her personality. The less toxins one accumulates in the subtle realm of mind and intelligence, the swifter one's mind will operate during training and daily activities.

9 a.m. or 9:30 a.m. to 2 p.m. or 3 p.m. This is a good time to perform work-related activities that culminate in a rich lunch composed of VP-friendly foods. If preparing for some event, whether a fight or show in the coming months, the VP type will do cardiovascular activities in the morning hours after eating a hearty breakfast (at least one and a half to two hours after breakfast). Assuming they have done some yoga already, a 30-minute run would suffice. The run could reflect some of the specifics they are working on, such as intervals of running, rope skipping, and shadow fighting.

The lunch should be eaten in a peaceful atmosphere, chewed slowly, and enjoyed. If no workout was performed in the morning (except for yoga stretches), then early lunch is preferable. If a workout was done after a good breakfast, then lunch can be eaten at noon or a little later. Since this is a time of increased fire in the atmosphere, a wise VP warrior will try to perform most of the important tasks of the day.

A martial arts event in the late morning or at around noon will be compatible with the VP constitution as long as a hearty breakfast was consumed earlier. A VP warrior will do fine eating a light lunch one and a half to two hours before the match.

The schedule can be adjusted in the following way: Performing morning yoga stretches and meditations but skipping the technical workout or cardio is a smart move, as is eating a more solid breakfast (if fighting before lunch). Ideally the competition event should happen before lunch when the warrior feels light yet fired up and his/her mind is sharp. Wise warriors do not exert themselves when hungry or thirsty.

A slower-pace, event-specific warm-up is good to avoid injury, as vatas possess great speed. For example, if a person is about to compete in semi-contact kumite (tae kwon do or kung-fu style) and strikes with full speed on a cold engine, some parts (tendons, muscles) may tear.

3:00 p.m. to 5:30 p.m. This time of the day is used for rejuvenation of life force and grounding. VP types will need at least some recovery time, as they have more delicate frameworks and edgy minds. Recommended activities include listening to pleasant sounds (nature or music), meditating, remaining in quietude for some time, taking a nap, and doing gentle yoga stretches. If more work remains to be done that day, a cup of VP-friendly tea would not be bad.

5:30 p.m. to 7:30 p.m. One does the remaining work of the day. One focuses on reflecting about today and planning ahead. An early supper composed of VP-recommended foods could be at 6 p.m. with friends and family.

7:30 p.m. to 10 p.m. Walking in the park or garden, watching tropical fish in a tank, or some other relaxing activity is good for the VP warrior. Breathing exercises meant to quiet the mind are to be performed at this time as well. Many VP types do well with aromas of essential oils or incense, which, when diffused in the room, can help adopt a certain mood.

Training for Vata-Kaphas

If you are primarily a fairly even combination of vata and kapha, then you must determine if the differences are more aligned physically (bone and muscle structure) or subtly (actions of mind, intellect).

If you are physically mostly a vata but your thinking and emotional patterns are of a kapha, then your nutrition should fulfill more the kapha nature, whereas your yoga practice should focus on harmonizing the vata aspects. Conversely, those with kapha body types and vata natures will eat more like vatas but do yoga according to kapha guidelines. With the change of seasons from late fall into early winter, one who is of dual nature will have to switch his/her focus from harmonizing vata (air) to harmonizing kapha (water).

Your unique body type will predispose you to overdoing things you think are good and right. You will greatly benefit from heat, as both vata (air, ether) and kapha (water, earth) lack the element of fire. That may manifest at the physical level as digestive issues and/or respiratory conditions. Sometimes you will lack energy and motivation to get going with your workout or day in general. You might be drawn to more peaceful forms of martial arts such as aikido and tai chi. However, to balance your body-mind system, it would be a good idea to practice a heat-increasing art like karate, although you may not feel like it is quite your element.

Karate, tae kwon do, and kickboxing will make you more assertive and determined in life in general. Breathing techniques that improve fire and circulation should be your mainstay, such as those for Prana, Vyana, Samana, and Apana Vayus (see five types of Chi). The strengths of your character may be sensitivity, modesty, ability to adapt, and respect for others.

5:15 a.m. to 6:15 a.m. This is the ideal wake-up time for a VK warrior. It is very important to begin his/her day by rising promptly after awakening to take a warm and even hot shower (in the wintertime). Scraping the tongue of toxins accumulated overnight and drinking one to two cups of warm lemon water will ignite their digestion gradually. Cleansing the nasal passages via the neti pot will ensure that their breathing and thinking during stretching practice will be maximized. Alternate-nostril breathing is recommended to balance you out. Placing vata- and kapha-controlling oils on the body, such as high-quality sesame oil (vata) or mustard oil (kapha), is recommended.

6:15 a.m. to 7:30 a.m. Powerful yoga postures to be implemented include, for the less flexible fighters, runner's lunge, wall push, power chair pose, triangle pose, warrior I, boat pose, child's pose, staff pose, head-to-knee pose, hero pose, and alligator twists. For the more flexible fighters, the following can be added: extended side angle pose, warrior III, intense back extension pose, upward single leg forward bend, full shoulder stand, unsupported cobra, reclining hero pose, and open legs forward bend. For very flexible fighters, additional poses are introduced such as revolving triangle, extended side angle pose, headstand, plow pose, and revolving head-to-knee pose.

The stretching practice should take at least close to 45 minutes and be followed by more specific breathing techniques such as the right-nostril breathing, which increases vital fires in the body. Right-nostril breathing is recommended if you are feeling either inertia (excess ether and/or earth) or agitation (excess air).

The morning time before breakfast is a great time to focus on technique-oriented movements. After doing yoga, the martial artist can do their forms, hone on single techniques, and do a few sets of energy-stabilizing stances or techniques such as the horse rider stance, simple kicks, and punches. The session should leave one feeling grounded and fired up

7:30 a.m. to 8:30 a.m. A medium-sized breakfast will consist of VK-friendly foods. It is important to consume breakfast quietly without unnecessary chatter while focusing on chewing. Digestion starts in the mouth, and since VK individuals do not have strong digestion, this instruction is of prime importance.

8:30 a.m. to 2 p.m. This is a good time to perform work-related activities that culminate in a rich lunch composed of VK-friendly foods. If preparing for some event, whether a fight or show in the coming months, the VK warrior will do cardiovascular activities in the morning hours after eating a hearty breakfast (at least one and a half to two hours after breakfast). Assuming they have done some yoga already, a 30-minute run would suffice. The run could reflect some of the specifics they are working on, such as intervals of running and rope skipping, shadow fighting

The lunch should be eaten in a peaceful atmosphere, chewed slowly, and enjoyed. If no workout was performed in the morning (except for yoga stretches), then an early lunch is preferable. If a workout was done after a good breakfast, then lunch can be eaten at noon or a little later. Since this is a time of increased fire in the atmosphere, a wise VK warrior will try to perform most of the important tasks of the day.

A martial arts event in the late morning or at around noon will be compatible with the cold aspect of the VK constitution as long as a hearty breakfast was consumed earlier. One could get away with eating a light lunch one and a half to two hours before the match.

The schedule can be adjusted in the following way: Performing morning yoga stretches and meditations but skipping the technical workout or cardio is a smart move, as is eating a more solid breakfast (if fighting before lunch). Ideally the competition event should happen before lunch when the warrior feels light yet fired up and his/her mind is sharp. Wise warriors do not exert themselves when hungry or thirsty.

A slower-pace, event-specific warm-up is good to avoid injury. For example, if a person is about to compete in semi-contact kumite (tae kwon do or kung-fu style) and strikes with full speed on a cold engine, some parts (tendons, muscles) may tear.

2 p.m. to 5 p.m. This time of the day is used for rejuvenation of life force and grounding. VK warriors require more recovery time, as they have more delicate frameworks and edgy minds. Recommended activities include listening to pleasant sounds (nature or music), meditating, remaining in quietude for some time, taking a nap, and doing gentle yoga stretches. If more workremains to be done that day, a cup of vata- or kapha-friendly tea would not be a good idea.

5 p.m. to 7 p.m. This time is for the remaining work of the day. The focus is on reflecting about today and planning ahead. An early supper composed of VK-recommended foods could be at 6 p.m. with friends and family.

7 p.m. to 10 p.m. Walking in the park or garden or doing some other relaxing activity is good for the VK constitution at this time. Breathing exercises meant to quiet the mind are to be performed at this time as well. Many VKs do well with aromas of essential oils or incense, which, when diffused in the room, can help adopt a certain mood.

Training for Pitta-Kaphas

If you are primarily a fairly even combination of pitta and kapha, then you must determine if the differences are more aligned physically (bone and muscle structure) or subtly (actions of mind, intellect).

If you are physically mostly a pitta but your thinking and emotional patterns are of a kapha, then your nutrition should fulfill more the kapha nature, whereas your yoga practice should focus on harmonizing the pitta aspects. Conversely, those with kapha body types and pitta natures will eat more like pittas but do yoga according to kapha guidelines.

With the change of seasons from spring to summer, one who is of dual nature will have to switch his/her focus from harmonizing kapha (water) to harmonizing pitta (fire)

As a PK, you will usually have the greatest level of overall muscular strength but have to be cautious not to overheat. You will have a limited ability to endure heat combined with moisture/humidity. You are both physically heavy and intense, which is a great asset to a martial artist, and to many athletes, for that matter. As you lack ether and air (vata), you may lack adaptability and, at the physical level, flexibility. Variegated workout routines that are both challenging and creative are the best way to harmonize your unique body type, along with certain types of breathing such as the ones increasing Prana, Vyana, and Apana Vayus.

5 a.m. to 6 a.m. This is the ideal wake-up time for a PK warrior. It is very important to begin his/her day by rising promptly after awakening to take a warm or cool shower (winter/summer). Scraping the tongue of toxins accumulated overnight and drinking one cup of cool lemon water will ignite their digestion gradually. Cleansing the nasal passages via the neti pot will ensure that their breathing and thinking during stretching practice will be maximized. This is the perfect time to do the alternate-nostril breathing, as well if still feeling lethargy or inertia. Placing fire-enhancing oils on the body, such as high quality mustard oil in the winter time and coconut oil in the spring and summer, is recommended.

6 a.m. to 7:30 a.m. Yoga postures for one's dual type will combine asanas from both the pitta and kapha regimens. One will need cooling postures in the spring and summer and heating ones in the winter. The stretching practice should take at least 30 minutes and be followed by more specific breathing techniques such as the right-nostril breathing, which increases vital fires in the body.

If preparing for some event, whether a fight or show in the coming months, the PK warriors will do intense cardiovascular activities in the morning hours before eating a very light breakfast. Pushing hard during the cardio sessions will set their energy right for most of the day. Assuming they have done some yoga already, a 45-minute run would suffice. The run could reflect some of the specifics they are working on, such as intervals of running and rope skipping, shadow fighting and even pushing tires, pulling sleds, and throwing heavy medicine balls.

The morning time before breakfast is also a great time to focus on technique-oriented movements. After doing yoga, the martial artist can do their forms, but in addition to honing on single techniques, as is often the traditional martial arts practice, they can do a few hundred of a variety of techniques. The session should leave one feeling fired up and ready to seize the day.

7:30 a.m. to 8:30 a.m. A small-sized breakfast will consist of PK-friendly foods. It is also advised that PK warriors skip breakfast entirely or just drink a glass of green juice consisting of PK-friendly foods, which would stir up their latent energies. That should be the case only in the colder seasons of the year.

8:30 a.m. to 3 p.m. This is a good time to perform work-related activities.

If there is a martial arts event in the late morning or at around noon that the warrior participates in, then the schedule can be adjusted in the following way: Performing morning yoga stretches and meditations but skipping the technical workout or cardio is a smart move, as is eating a more solid breakfast. Wise warriors do not exert themselves when hungry or thirsty. Ideally the competition event should happen before lunch when the warrior feels light yet fired up and his/her mind is sharp.

PK warriors will need a somewhat intense event-specific warm-up before. They need to spend more time igniting the fire in the winter season. For example, performing combinations of technically easy punches and kicks with 70 percent power for 10 to 15 minutes with short breaks in between sets would be all right. Such a warm-up might even feel like a workout to a vata or pitta, but a PK warrior will oftentimes feel good about it.

3 p.m. to 4:30 p.m. This is a good time for a hearty lunch consisting of pitta- or kapha-friendly articles.

4:30 p.m. to 7:30 p.m. Since the ether and air elements are prevalent in the atmosphere at this time, PK warriors could use it to perform the hardest tasks of their jobs. This will give them the extra wind they do not have in the morning or evening hours. It is also a good idea to drink some spicy tea to accelerate the surge of energy. An appropriate time for that is 4:30 p.m. to 5 p.m.

Because the fire element is still present but slowly decreasing after 2 p.m. and the air and ether elements are rising in influence, a time range between 2 p.m. and 4 p.m. would a very good time for PKs to compete. A shorter and less intense warm-up might suffice. At that time, the air and ether are completing the PK warrior's weaker spots. In contrast, when PKs compete in the morning, they may still lack the functional principle of mobility. And when they compete in the late afternoon, although the light energy of air and ether will still be present, the earth and water elements and the mode of ignorance will already be building up.

7:30 p.m. to 8:30 p.m. This is time for a light dinner with friends and family.

8:30 p.m. to 10:00 p.m. The PK warrior will perform somewhat intense pitta- and kapha-specific yoga poses or even a light group martial arts practice. Sometimes PKs will require a more intense practice in the evening that will not overstimulate or tire them to the same degree as it would a V or VP warrior. It must be remembered, though, that dinner time and quantity should be adjusted—such as by eating earlier or by cutting portions in half—to allow two hours for at least the first stage of digestion to occur. The yoga practice, workout, or martial arts practice should not last past 10 p.m.

10 p.m. to 10:30 p.m. One can relax and perform some evening meditation. The PK warrior should go to sleep shortly after.

A Sample Karate-Based Workout for the Vata Constitution

For demos of the following workouts visit our website, CompleteWarriorFitness.com.

It is a humid and somewhat hot late morning with the temperature about 85 degrees Fahrenheit. The sky is somewhat cloudy, but you can feel the scorching rays piercing through. Fire and water energies are ruling the sky. They should assist you a great deal today since you want to zero in on power hand strikes in your backyard. Knowing what workout lies ahead of you, after your morning meditation, you stretched, especially your lower back and arms, and applied strengthening oils to your arms and legs. You also had a decent meal at around 7 a.m., and now the energy is kicking in. Just now, you performed five rounds of both the Ujjayi and Vyana Vayu breathing with special focus on channeling the Prana force to your arms and hands.

You take off your sandals and walk up to two giant trees that have Japanese *makiwaras* (karate striking boards) plastered to them. You look at them carefully and begin your warm-up sequence.

Sequence 1

Repeat once in a circuit-like fashion as a warm-up.

1. 10 karate-style push-ups on grass, slow tempo, with full range of motion. Arms and elbows are positioned close to the sides of the body, the hands are clenched in hard fists, in a neutral position (palms facing each other). The upper body weight is resting on the first two knuckles of each hand. As you lower your upper body, the chin should almost touch the floor. 30-second break.
2. 15 suspended sit-ups (legs are positioned up and head is down) using a chin-up bar or bracing the legs around partner's hips. Take a 30-second break.
3. 10 karate-style push-ups on concrete, medium tempo with high range of motion. 15-second break.
4. 10 torso rotations to the right and left with band attached to door knob or handle. 30-second break.
5. 10 karate-style push-ups on concrete, fast tempo with a shortened range of motion. 30-second break.

Sequence 2

Repeat once in a circuit-like fashion as a warm-up.

1. 10 explosive karate push-ups on concrete. Use a shortened range of motion. 15- to 30-second break.
2. 10 torso rotations to the right and left with band attached to door handle, fast tempo. 30-second break.
3. 10 single-armed triceps push-offs on incline bench or surface (simplified one-armed push-ups), right and left. 45-second break.
4. 10 medium-force strikes to the *makiwara* from either the *zenkutsu-dachi* (forward long lunge stance) or the regular split fighting stance (square stance with both knees slightly bent). Perform the punches from both leads (left- and right-foot lead). Use the traditional *seiken chudan-tsuki* (fore-fist straight punch) technique from a guard-up position, and you will be striking with the same knuckles you used for push-ups. In boxing, this striking will be called a "cross" since you will punch with your rear hand. 30-second break.

Sequence 3

Repeat at least two or three times in a circuit-like fashion.

1. 10 explosive strikes to the *makiwara* from *migi zenkutsu-dachi* (right forward long stance). 15-second break.

2. 10 explosive strikes to the *makiwara* from *hidari zenkutsu-dachi* (left forward long stance).
   15-second break.
3. 20 explosive strikes from the right lead stance.
   10-second break.
4. 20 explosive strikes from the left lead stance.
   30-second break.

Sequence 4

Repeat at least two or three times in a circuit-like fashion.

1. 5 explosive strikes from the left lead stance.
   10-second break.
2. 5 explosive strikes from the right lead stance.
   30-second break.
3. 10 medium force strikes from the left lead stance, but cross-jab style. Right (rear) hand punches first and then immediately the left follows. 30-second break.
4. 10 medium force strikes from the right lead stance, but cross-jab style. Left (rear) hand punches first and then immediately the right follows. 30-second break.
5. 5 explosive strikes from the left lead, same as above but with more power. 10-second break.
6. 5 explosive strikes from the right lead. 30-second break.

As you may notice, in this type of workout, the focus is placed on a very specific warm-up. The first two sequences basically constitute a warm-up. Sequences 3 and 4 are the training proper. One should not repeat the warm-up sequences more than once (unless one is cold and the environment is cold), but one should repeat sequences 3 and 4 as many times as desired.

A Sample Karate-Based Workout for the Pitta Constitution

For demos of the following workouts visit our website, CompleteWarriorFitness.com.

It is early spring and the weather is somewhat humid because there was some rain a couple days ago. Today the temperature is about 55 to 60 degrees Fahrenheit with a little breeze. The sky is cloudy. The time is about 3 p.m., and the air and ether energies are ruling the sky. They should support you well today since you want to focus on cardiovascular work. You did your morning meditation already as well as your stretching, especially for your legs and hips. You also had a sturdy meal at around noon, and now the energy is kicking in. You still needed to perform the right-nostril breathing to stir up the fire element. One minute was sufficient.

You grab a jump rope and shove it in the pocket of your jacket. Then you put on your ninja shoes so it feels like you're running barefoot.

Sequence 1

Repeat once in a circuit-like fashion as a warm-up.

1. 1 medium pace lap around the block, for a 1/4 mile.
2. Skip rope fast for 30 seconds.
3. Shadow fight with focus on *mae-geri* (front kicks), *yoko-geri* (side kicks), *ushiro-geri* (back kicks), non-traditional *seiken chudan-tsuki* (straight punches with guard up), *shita* (uppercuts), and some *soto-uke* (shortened inside blocks). About a 1-minute duration at medium pace.

Sequence 2

Repeat once in a circuit-like fashion as a warm-up.

1. 1 faster pace lap around the block.
2. Skip rope fast for 30 seconds.
3. More intense shadow fight with focus on *mawashi-geri gedan* (low kicks), *mawashi-geri* (mid hook kicks), *ushiro-geri* (back kicks), uppercuts, and hooks. 1-minute duration.

Sequence 3

Repeat two or three times in a circuit-like fashion.

1. 1 lap around the block of sprint/jog intervals.
2. Kangaroo jumps for 30 seconds.
3. High jump squats for 15 seconds.

4. Intense shadow fight with focus on *uchi-kaege* (round crescent kicks), *hiza-geri* (knee kicks), and *mawashi-geri gedan* (low kicks). 1-minute duration.

Sequence 4

Repeat once in a circuit-like fashion.

1. Slower pace jog around the block for 1 lap. Walk the last 100 feet while breathing in deeply, holding for a moment, and exhaling air dynamically through the mouth. This kind of breathing will restore Prana in the mind (as the brain may get a little dull after a strenuous workout) and help release the excessive fire element that rose to the surface of the body due to exertion.
2. Slow shadow fight with simple techniques, purposefully slowed down. Perform defensive techniques (blocks) such as abbreviated *uchi-uke* (outer midsection), *soto-uke* (inside midsection), *gedan-barai* (outer low), *jodan-uke* (outer high). Hold many kicks for a half or full second to emphasize the landing aspect of every technique.

As you may suppose, the number of sequences in this workout may vary depending on whether you are working on anaerobic endurance (shorter duration/high intensity as in a karate bout) or aerobic endurance (longer duration/lighter intensity as in a soccer game).

A Sample Karate-Based Workout for the Kapha Constitution

For demos of the following workouts visit our website, CompleteWarriorFitness.com.

The weather is somewhat hot and humid with a little summer breeze. The temperature is about 90 degrees Fahrenheit. The time is about 5:30 a.m. The air and ether energies are ruling the sky. However, the humidity factor seems to neutralize much of it. Your plan is to focus on power, which is a combination of strength and speed. You did your morning meditation already as well as your stretching, focusing especially on your arms and chest to facilitate Udana Vayu flow. To optimize metabolism, you did not eat anything yet and made sure to take some spicy tea to wake you up more. When you came outside and assessed the environment, the grass still had some pleasant dew droplets on it. You took off your shoes and stepped on it to perform the much-needed right-nostril breathing. There was still some stagnation in your mind, probably because you ran out of time to complete your morning stretching. Therefore, you resorted to a few minutes of Udana and Vyana Vayu breathing to stir up the fire element. After five minutes, you began to feel the right kind of power.

The tractor tire is there standing next to the giant tree, as you and your training partner left it there a few days ago. Today it is only you though.

Sequence 1

Repeat two or three times in a circuit-like fashion as a warm-up.

1. 15 jumping jacks.
2. 15 burpees.
3. 15 push-ups with torso rotation on one hand.
4. Lift tire overhead and drop. 10 reps.

Sequence 2

Repeat two or three times in a circuit-like fashion.

1. Lift tire overhead and drop. 10 reps.
2. Straddle tire, and ground and pound (30 seconds, non-stop action). Heavy bag gloves are suggested. 1 rep.
3. Sprint and jump over a stack of mattresses or a box (cardboard or Styrofoam) in a tiger jump to roll in a defensive fall (use of padded mat suggested).
4. 5 explosive punches to shield (held by partner) or to heavy bag positioned by the tree.
5. 5 explosive *hiza-geri* (knee kicks) to shield.
6. 5 fast *mawashi-geri gedan* (low kicks) to shield.

Sequence 3

Repeated two or three times in a circuit-like fashion.

1. 5 explosive *shita* (alternating uppercuts) to pads.

2. 1 power push.
3. 5 explosive *mawashi-geri gedan* (low kicks) to shields. 5 reps on each side.
4. 5 explosive hammer strikes while kneeling on the heavy bag. Perform 5 consecutive strikes, then switch to the other side.

In this particular workout, in addition to a traditional mixed-martial arts approach, there is an element of acrobatics that kaphas might enjoy and greatly benefit from. It will expand their energy outward and make them more interactive, assertive, and energized in daily life. It is, indeed, a very good way to boost their metabolism for the rest of the day. Of course, as a general note, other body types may want to, like to, and need to try opposite approaches to training. For example, a pitta would try to do a kapha's workout for the simple reason that they are preparing for a tournament that involves level changes (from kicking to striking to a takedown). That is fine and perfect, but someone who tries a workout approach that does not suit their body type or, better yet, that will tend to throw them off their harmony long term, must take extra caution to guard their physical (body) and subtle system (mind and five Vayus) from overexertion.

Recovery is as important or more important than training itself is, and there is not much benefit in pushing to your maximum if you are not able to recover sufficiently from any kind of training, especially the training that ultimately throws you off your unique state of harmony.

Other Workout Routines for Warriors

If you are engaged in martial arts, you will have to train for muscular endurance, usually with high anaerobic component. In other words, you will need to sustain intermittent quick bursts of energy that will last from 10 minutes to an hour. The following workouts will prepare you for that. For full demos, visit our website, CompleteWarriorFitness.com.

The Wonderful 7

The Wonderful 7 features seven different exercises for major muscle groups. Repeat each 54 times before you move on to the next exercise.
1. Push-ups. Progression: Alternating-push-ups.
2. Crunches. Progression: Jackknives or hanging-from-bar leg lifts.
3. Dumbbell clean and press. Progression: The same but on one leg.
4. Band curls with superband. Progression: The same but standing on a Bosu Ball.
5. Horizontal dips. Progression: Vertical dips.
6. Burpies. Progression: Single-legged burpies.
7. Back kicks. Progression: Alternating to focus mitt.

The Magic 18

The Magic 18 features 18 different exercises for various muscle groups, each repeated for one minute non-stop. It is important not to stop for 18 minutes. Your only break happens when you transition between the exercises. After 18 minutes of non-stop work, you can take a two-minute break and begin round two (optional).

1. Walk sideways push-ups.
2. TRX or medium cable rows.
3. Crunches.
4. Side step on Bosu ball and double straight punch with dumbbell.
5. Front kicks in the air.
6. Prone position (flat on stomach) forward punches (feet off the floor).
7. Crouching tiger kicks (crouch position and alternating back kick).
8. Jump around a heavy bag and slap it.
9. Plank.
10. Alternating jumping lunges.
11. Intense back extension.
12. Alternating dumbbell military press.
13. Alternating torso rotations with band attached to a pole or cable station.
14. Prone position torso rotation on hands (hold yourself up on one hand each time you switch).
15. Karate cracker squat (sit on each foot with the other leg extended to the side, and switch).
16. Skip rope.
17. Kangaroo jumps (jumps in a completely squatted position, sitting on your heels).

18. Stepper jumps (both feet land on the platform and, when jumping off, on the floor).

The Lucky 108

The Lucky 108 features eight different exercises. A warrior repeats each exercise 108 times before he/she moves to the next one. The workout is timed so that the faster one does it, the higher one's level of anaerobic endurance.

1. Walk sideways push-ups with leg lift on each one. Progression: jump sideways and perform such a push-up.
2. Alternating bent over lunges (round your back and reach to your foot each time you lunge).
3. Chin-ups (bar or assisted with an elastic band).
4. Alternating crescent kicks (knee straight, also called "round" kicks).
5. Leg lifts or knee-ups while holding onto chin-up bar.
6. Alternating dumbbell straight punches while sidestepping.
7. Defensive fallback to get up and hook kick. (Make sure to use a well-padded mat)
8. Hyperextensions on hyperextension bench.

Chapter VII

Important Variables for Each Constitution

Frequency of Training

Volume-wise, kaphas are capable of and should do the most physical work with minimal but specific recovery time. They could even do multiple workouts per day with varying intensities. Vatas will grow and benefit the most from less volume in general. However, intensity must be there to enhance performance. Vatas require the most recovery time to perform at their best, especially beginners. Pittas stand in the middle. Intermediate- and advanced-level trainees of a pitta body type will greatly benefit from short bursts of very intense workouts, let's say an all-out, heavy bag drill of 15 minutes repeated every other day with some technical changes. In between, they will do other types of skill and strength work as necessary per their goals.

There certainly are standards more or less established and confirmed by "in trench" experience of coaches when it comes to volume of work necessary for athletes of certain sport disciplines, combat arts not being an exception. However, it would be a sensible idea to assign work volume based on individuals' body types rather than other factors. That would protect the athlete from draining his/her system and, for example, succumbing to a flu. That would be healthy and save the athlete's valuable life energy (which would otherwise be used for coping with the flu).

Seasonal Training

Obviously, most martial arts disciplines require a substantial amount of fiery energy (in the context of this work, pitta). I would even call karate or kick-boxing a pitta discipline. All body types do contain some pitta, just as they do have the other two types of energies in them (vata, kapha). To make the pitta type of discipline benefit the athlete the most, it could be performed in a pitta-friendly season (a cooler and dryer season) and at a pitta-friendly time of day (early morning). That would ensure that the participant or practitioner feels his/her best and does not disharmonize/disorient his/her energies.

Another approach that functions well for external performance is to practice a pitta discipline in a pitta-aggravating environment (hot and humid) to unleash the aggressive pitta aspect during competition. Match that with someone who is of a purer pitta constitution and you have a raging tiger in the ring. In the context of earlier sections of this work, I would re-emphasize the importance of pitta-friendly recovery, which may take longer in such a situation. Whether one's state of mind is clear and optimal during such an imbalanced situation is highly doubtful. Therefore, the Ayurvedic recommendation is that each body type practices disciplines, or at least the right yoga regimens, that balance their individual constitutions rather than necessarily produce numbers.

As far as vata types are concerned, their state of balance is enhanced by performing less complex, slower, and more static exercises and disciplines such as strength training with weights, isometrics, swimming, or tai chi. Pittas would do well practicing in more vata- or kapha-like conditions, including vata or kapha times of day, seasons, and, ultimately, vata and/or kapha types of disciplines (tai chi). And conversely, kapha individuals will do the best for their constitutions if they embrace fiery and fast disciplines such as wing-chun, boxing, or tae kwon do. Whether they are successful in the eyes of others and produce numbers is a secondary consideration, the priority being to preserve one's unique margin of health and happiness.

Type of Training

For the best balancing of someone with a vata constitution, one should choose arts that increase primarily the fiery and watery energy, which would definitely include karate, kickboxing, and some harder styles of kung fu (that resemble karate). The watery energy would be increased by arts like tai chi, qigong, and certain yogic asanas, as well as by heating forms of breathing. Arts that are very complex and rely on speed would allow vatas who practice them to excel but would ultimately contribute to throwing them off their constitutional balance.

For the ultimate balancing of someone with a pitta constitution, one should choose arts that promote sensitivity of touch and adaptability of movements that do not stir up the innate and already dominant fire element. For example, the often-prone-to-anger-and-aggression pitta warrior will cool down more by practicing "sticky hands" in the wing chun academy or by practicing aikido than by jumping into kickboxing or karate training, which all too often rely on hardness and rigidity of techniques. Practicing karate with zeal would more likely make a pitta an overly strict, stern, and controlling individual at the emotional level, but no doubt a pitta would love that kind of practice since it would focus and increase the powers he is already in possession of. Assuming that such a pitta would begin the karate practice, he/she should at least balance it out by swimming a few times a week to cool off and/or practice a cooling form of yoga asana and breathing.

For the optimal balancing of a kapha constitution, a warrior should choose arts that promote air, ether, and fire: arts that rely on speed, quick transitions of movements, lightness, explosive movements such as tae kwon do, softer kung-fu styles, mixed-martial arts, jujitsu, karate, etc. Kaphas may not be the fastest practitioners of those arts or the elite of their group, but such arts are sure more likely to balance their constitutions than slow and gentle arts. A kapha who nevertheless chooses less dynamic arts would still do great adding some explosive and dynamic types of exercise to their workout regimen.

As you can see, it is not about which art is better in and of itself but about which is more suitable for the warrior's constitutional type. Once the art is chosen by a warrior, he/she must know what the psychological and physiological effects of such practice are so as to balance the unnecessary energies stimulated by such practice. Similarly, it is not about how many fast kicks one can throw or how hard one can punch but about how clear and strong one's mind remains in the midst of it.

Quick Ways to Replenish Lost Chi

The dissipation of the vital force occurs naturally in life and especially through physical and mental exertion, be it through a tough workout routine or giving a speech in which you transfer the energy to the audience. The force that is dissipated is specifically Prana Vayu, the master energy, and it is used up through Udana and Vyana Vayu. It is in our best interest to assess our daily levels of

Prana and, based on the daily schedule, optimize it the right way before and after the physical activity.

Assuming you are in a good mood and have good overall energy during your workout, you may feel great focus on the muscles at work, on the breathing, and on the objects that the energy is going into (for example, a heavy bag that's being punched and kicked). What happens is both a subtle and gross energy transfer (the bag is moving, the opponent is falling due to being struck by your force, the board is breaking). As you may remember from physics, for every action there is a reaction. In the world of practical (exoteric) and subtle (esoteric) combat art, there is a gross and subtle loss of energy for every punch you execute and for every *kiai* (warrior yell) you shout. Thus, after a good workout, you may feel your mind and brain slower and duller, as the mind has a tendency to get "stuck" on objects and images in the external realm. Your energy, due to an intense activity, is in the mode of outward flow, and you are, so to speak, "outside of yourself," which is the opposite of being centered. As the energy is directed externally, you must reverse it to begin replenishing the lost Prana lest you want to be weak and vulnerable for the rest of the day.

It is also common for us to catch a flu or cold after a strenuous workout, and we usually are not sure why, because we felt so strong coming into the workout. So here are some easy and practical ways to begin your Prana-rejuvenation process immediately following the activity as well as some ways to load up on Prana prior to an intense workout.

Popular approach:
Have a power drink of some sort, like a protein shake (to rebuild lean muscle), or a glass of homemade juice, or a rehydration drink (to replenish sugar and electrolyte levels in the blood).

Yoga approach:
Perform a cooling type of breathing such as left-nostril breathing to increase water and earth elements. Also, *ibuki* breathing would be great here, such as the front silent breath (see "Breathing Techniques in Traditional Karate" in chapter IV). Certain mudras, or hand positions, can be helpful, such as Prana mudra, Vayu mudra, or Prithivi mudra.

Isolation approach:
Remove yourself from a stimulating environment, and lie down with feet elevated, possibly in quietude. You can combine this strategy with massaging and pressing particular energy points on the body, such as the feet, upper back, neck, or any muscles that were heavily used in the workout. See the "Marma Points in the Martial Arts" section of chapter IV to choose the correct points.

Acupressure/massage approach:
Massage or press special points on the body that are

important energy centers, thus restoring optimal energy flow in the body-mind system.

Mega-C approach:
Load up on quality vitamin C before and immediately after your workout. Contrary to popular belief, studies have shown that a mega dose of at least 2,500 milligrams per day may be the amount needed by your immune system to fight off any viruses or bacteria around.[24]

All of the above-mentioned strategies can and should be combined to suit our purposes, which will reflect our preferences. For instance, after an anaerobic cardio workout such as the mixed-martial artists use, one could first of all drink 16 ounces of mint lemonade, take a contrast shower (use warm and cool water interchangeably), and stretch and massage the muscles that worked the most in a cool, quiet, and darkened room. In the restoration room, there could be an essential oil diffuser with eucalyptus oil to assist in taking deep breaths. After 15 to 20 minutes of such rejuvenation, one could take 25 grams of whey protein in the form of a shake, followed by a 30-minute catnap.

---

[24] Research based on Linus Pauling that is becoming confirmed by more and more findings today.

How to Balance External Factors versus Internal Factors with Your Training

By now you know a lot about your body type, the types of food that strengthen your inherent equilibrium, the types of yoga stances that can be incorporated into your regimen, and breathing techniques that all balance out your natural constitution. You also learned about the special points on the body (marmas) and sound vibrations (mantras) that can augment your mental harmony. You may recall that I talked about the forces of vata, pitta, and kapha existing in the external environment, from which they affect your own body-mind system. Recall "Three Energies in the External World" in chapter I. Knowing all these key factors to balancing your own constitution, you must decide now how to navigate the vehicle of your body and mind in the midst of miscellaneous external and internal factors that you perceive. The rule of thumb is to assess the following four factors in the right order:

1. **Your mental state.** How you feel, your emotional or psychological state, what you feel like doing as far as exercise. Do you feel like kicking the heavy bag, or do you feel like lifting heavy weights? Is your mind acting fast today or a little sluggish?
2. **Physical state.** How do you perceive the state of your muscles, tendons, joints, etc.? Are you still

sore in specific areas of the body from the previous workout? Are you bruised in certain spots due to sparring? Do your muscles feel tight and rigid? Do you feel warm or cold?

3. **Environmental factors.** This really matters if you train outdoors. If the workout is inside a gymnasium or dojo, you can skip through this. Is the weather hot and humid, or windy and dry? Is it raining? What time of the day is it? What season are we in?

4. **Your normally planned workout.** Are you due for a strength session (lifting weights) or skill training (karate technique)? Are you doing a group training with your partners, or an individual workout?

It is essential to consider the above factors in the order given before deciding what type of training to do. This is so because the workout that does not match your mental state will tend to throw off any or all of the five types of Chi for the rest of the day or longer. It is common to base our workouts strictly on the schedule given by our coach and our physical state. Therefore, mostly factors 2 and 4 are taken into consideration. The mental state and environment are given less, if any, weight in the attempted workout.

Let me give you a couple examples which demonstrate the importance of considering your mental state and environmental factors. The first example is from my own workout.

Example 1

Just a short half hour ago, my boss and I had a rough talk. Quickly thereafter, I walked out of the gym to face a dry summer lunchtime heat. Although it was my time to eat, I was not really hungry. The upper body and especially my head were full of accumulated energy that wished to be somehow freed up. The planned workout was with my sparring buddy at 2 p.m. till 3:30 p.m. in the forest area nearby. It was noon.

I quickly texted him to postpone our training till tomorrow. I drove home and took a cool shower, did some left-nostril breathing, and gave myself a head massage. Next, instead of coming out in the heat to do the workout, I stayed in my private training room that had a temperature of only 65 degrees. There I threw some punches to the *makiwara* and kicks to the heavy bag. I especially focused on channeling my energy into the target. After the dynamic 30-minute session, I performed 20 minutes of upper-body and mid-back stretches to release the upward moving air and pacify the fire element. The stretches I performed included the cat, runner's lunge, spread legs forward bend, head-to-knee pose, reclining hero pose, spinal twist, supine single hamstring stretch, etc. I made sure to exhale through the mouth at every stretch which has the potential of releasing more fiery energy from the system.[25] Next, I followed with another cool, short shower and a little marma point manipulation in the areas of the *stanarohita, hridaya, sthapani,* and *avarta* marmas (upper chest, heart region, forehead, eyebrows), all of which control the active elements of air, ether, and fire. All of that was done with mantra music in the background.

The result of my actions was that the already stirred up and accumulated emotions that included fire, air, and water were not allowed to grow via a more heated workout in the humid and hot environment at the time when fire is dominant. The excessively accumulated emotions were controlled and slowly released by the cooling actions of water, expressive exercise, cooling types of breathing, energy massage (marma points), and stretches. There was no denial of the energies nor further stimulation of them. I just let them peacefully leave the body-mind system so I could return to my normal state of being.

In terms of the elements, the hyper and fiery energy in the mind, which was heating up the whole system, and the hot conditions outside were neutralized by the coolness and slowness of water, yoga stretches, and breathing. The vehicles through which the excessive energies left were dynamic exercise that channeled them, proper stretches, and exhalation through the mouth. I had a good night's rest and was ready to take on another day when I woke up.

---

[25] Most physical yoga practice, asana, is done while breathing through the nose only.

Example 2

Sebastian had a long day at work that ended after 7 p.m. on this Wednesday. His mind was tired, and he was already kind of sluggish. He remembered, though, how in the morning he was really excited about the karate training at 7:30 p.m. Well, not anymore. But Sebastian has always had a big heart. He did not want to let his friends down, what to speak of his master instructor, whom he even admired. He already paid for his monthly training anyway. As a proactive person, Sebastian already had his workout bag in the car and quickly drove up to the karate dojo, right on the nose. He did not mind missing his supper. Hastily, he changed his clothes and ran into the training hall. The preliminary ritual of meditating, bowing down, and reciting the warrior oath had already started, so Sebastian sat in the corner kneeling and waited for them to finish. As was the custom, after the preliminary ritual, the master came up to him and ordered him to do 100 push-ups for coming late. Then Sebastian was able to join the group for a hard technique-oriented karate workout that lasted until 9 p.m.

During the course of the workout, Sebastian's mind was off, and he could not quickly assimilate the instructor's comments. His determination was forced upon the mind. Even though his heart was pounding due to physical exertion, his mind remained mostly dull, and it seemed like it did not want to follow the body. By the end of the grueling training session, Sebastian was utterly exhausted even though sparring bouts had two opponents less than usual. He felt little energy to talk to his training buddies, and he was even ticked off when one of them mentioned something jokingly about Sebastian being slow today. Sebastian hated when others pointed out his weaknesses. He barely dragged himself into his car and went home. His wife gave him a questioning and disappointed look and pointed to the table with food on it. "It's cold by now. The kids are fast asleep." She did not say anything more, and he did not feel like talking.

The next morning Sebastian overslept, rushed to work again, missed breakfast, was pulled over by the police for speeding, and was even more late for work. That set him off on a bad vibe for the rest of the day. He did not like when things did not go exactly according to his plan. At work, Sebastian seemed more aggressive toward and less understanding of his colleagues and even his customers.

In this example, we can appreciate how a strict adherence to a plan or routine does not always support our harmonious existence. Sure, Sebastian might have felt good to be able to checkmark his workout for the day, but then he missed many other marks afterward. His excessive zeal to be able to fulfill his workout obligations burned up his energy completely to the point that his energy deficit transferred into the next day. Sebastian's fire was not pacified, because he worked out hard in the evening, ate late, and could not fall asleep. He also did not wake up properly the next day, missed his breakfast the next day, and tried to do things fast, all the while striving to match everything to his demanding schedule. The elements of fire and air were overly dominant. As a result, they depleted his earth and water elements, which provide a sense of self-satisfaction, groundedness, and peace. No effort was made to counteract this fiery momentum, and in the long run, Sebastian was not making himself nor anyone else around him happy.

The quick and commonsense solution to this situation was to simply not attend his evening workout, make it home in time for supper, see his wife and kids, and get a good night's rest. The next day would certainly be better and the following day, Sebastian would be rested and his mindset would be right for a great karate workout.

When the Pot Is Already Boiling

In the course of martial arts training and maintaining your natural harmony, you may sometimes still find yourself overflowing with energies/emotions that are not your true self. Take, for instance, a situation where someone says something negative to you and you, although feeling angry, smile and say something nice to the person. You did great. On another occasion, a similar situation occurs, and the anger within you does not even arise. Excellent. On another day, when a similar event happens, you quickly retaliate with some angry remark. These three responses exemplify how you are in decent, perfect, and out-of-harmony states. This can be illustrated by an example of a water-filled pot on the stove.

You are trying to warm-up the water so that it is neither hot or cold, just warm. You expertly turn the electric stove on and wait a minute or two until the water reaches the desired temperature. When the desired temperature is reached, you turn off the stove or take the pot off of it. However, at times you may get busy with something else, leave the pot unattended, and not come back in time. When you hear the boiling water splashing out of the pot and onto the hot stove surface, you are immediately alarmed. You rush to the stove, quickly take the pot off the stove, and turn the stove off to prevent further water spillage. Then turn the stove off.

Your actions and reactions in both instances are effective, but their order is different because of the difference in the water temperature. As this example shows, we have to act differently depending on how much out of balance our energies become. By the proper execution of your body-type and mental-type regimen, by keeping your focus on the inner kingdom, you will probably never reach the point of overspilling of your energies when you act angry, frustrated, depressed, etc. All you will need to do is gently steer to the left or right by adjusting the foods, breathing techniques, etc.

When, however, you are in a habit of neglecting and overlooking some things for an extended time, the point of overflow will come, and then you will have to release the excessive energies in a less destructive and, therefore, still positive way. For example, when someone says something negative to me, I get angry and say something in retaliation. Then, rather than quarreling with the person, I will stop talking to the person (take the pot off the stove) and quickly drive to the nearby gym to engage in an intense kick-boxing workout (direct the spilled water to some dry cloth). That would replace the reaction of even punching the person who offended me (as I already said something bad to them).

Sample Scenarios for Coaches

Scenario 1: John Bereck

John is naturally a 140-pound kickboxer but for different reasons he fights at 155 pounds. He puts a lot of energy into maintaining his higher unnatural weight during training, especially in the days preceding the weigh-in. After the competition, he loses quite a few pounds, relaxes for a couple weeks, and starts the cycle of training and re-gaining weight. He puts in a weekly total of 30 hours of training (skill, cardio, strength, plyometrics). He feels heavier and slower than in his college years, and he has a hard time becoming a pro, but he is doing fairly well anyway. His coaches are on his case to get his game up to the next level, and that creates a great amount of stress for him.

Optimizing John's situation: First of all, there is the problem of excessive stress. The coaches demand something from him that is very hard to obtain from the platform that John is situated at. John is artificially situated at the higher body weight, which keeps oscillating due to frequent competition. The much higher weight that he must maintain most of the year thwarts John's natural speed and agility of movement, and its all-too-often oscillations force the vata (air, ether) elements out of balance. Sure, a slightly heavier weight for a vata body type is fine because it adds to bone strength, protects the inner organs more, and increases confidence levels. However, the 15-pound increase is too huge of a difference to maintain most of the year. Thus, John and his coaches would be smart to place him in a lighter division where he would be able to exhibit his full warrior features such as speed, agility, etc. That would reduce John's stress to a healthy level. He would also do well to decrease his workout time to about four days a week, two to three hours a day, with each workout day further divided into two or three shorter sessions. All of that would make his training time more energetic, focused, meaningful, and, therefore, effective. John would almost always be fully rested and at his best.

Scenario 2: Jessica Cronmick

Jessica is naturally a 150-pound *judoka* (a person who practices the art of judo), but she competes at 125 pounds. For much of the year, she maintains such a low and lean weight, except for a month or two. Jessica puts in about 20 hours of total practice per week. She is very successful in her discipline of competition, one of the reasons being her sturdier bone structure, whereas most of her opponents keep a lighter weight in daily life. She enjoys the career but does not feel great most of the year. Jessica hates gaining weight during the off-season and worries about what everyone else will think of her, but that's when her body actually feels rested. Jessica feels like she will give it all up one day and just walk away to do something completely different.

Optimizing Jessica's situation: First of all, there is the problem of Jessica's feeling fulfilled in her profession. Whether she should indeed look for another career is beyond the subject matter of this book. The lack of satisfaction may simply be due to the fact that Jessica is forced to maintain unnaturally low weight most of the year. It seems that demands on her body are taking effect on her mind. Forcing the unnatural body weight certainly has such a psychological effect. A smart strategy for Jess would be to simply fight at 145 or 155 pounds and work out more to maintain explosiveness and quickness at the heavier weight. An increased workout time of 30 hours per week would ensure that lean muscle is added on more than body fat is. During the off-season, Jessica would not be gaining or losing much weight. Thus, the psychological burden of gaining weight would be eliminated once she accepted herself at 145 to 150 pounds. The off-season would be far more enjoyable with a variety of engagements such as biking, canoeing, and fitness boot camps but with a decrease in training volume to about 20 hours.

Scenario 3: Phil Bartos

Phil has been a naturally 170-pound amateur boxer competing at 165 pounds for the past five years without much success. Most of the time he does great in training, putting in at least five hours of light to heavy sparring per week and a total of 40 hours of total training. He is getting a little older now, but the coaches are pushing him to eat more and train more if he is to achieve the pro level. Time is short, they say, and stakes are high. Phil feels physically strong during training and sparring but emotionally discontented. When he is in the ring, he has a hard time clearing his mind to follow the strategy that his instructors give him. Phil then loses his focus more or less during the fight and allows fear of failure to rule his heart.

Optimizing Phil's situation: In this scenario, it looks like Phil could benefit from either reevaluating his training goals or adopting some meditational techniques specific to his mental nature. Training more and eating more are not likely to get Phil over his sticking point, since the blockage seems to be on the subtle, mental plane.

Chapter VIII

The Complete Warrior Gym Facility

To properly fulfill the meaning of this work and facilitate harmonious training of combat athletes, the following gymnasium design is proposed. It will ensure the polishing of the three types of armor that every sincere combat athlete should possess.

There are three training halls in each facility: the general fitness hall, martial arts hall, and yoga hall. The general fitness hall is the first one sees. To the left is the martial arts hall. To the right, the yoga hall. The three gyms can be on three floors as well, but a flat area is preferred since the roof can be opened for fresh air during a hard workout or, weather permitting, anytime.

General Fitness Hall—Physical Armor

This hall is accessible to members who look for general fitness as well as martial artists who like to complement their specific training with some strength training or added cardiovascular training. The music played in this room is a general type of music, but it is closer to a meditational type. This hall would more likely resemble a typical fitness gym and would consist of

- a few elliptical machines;
- free weights, like kettlebells and such, along with a few flat adjustable benches to modify exercises;
- medicine balls, stability balls, and Bosu balls;
- platforms for step-ups;
- an adjustable cable station;
- a pull-up/dip station;
- a stretching area.

Martial Arts Hall—Physical Armor

This hall is accessible to members who look for general martial arts training and to expand their expertise in that direction. The music played in this studio is a harder and more upbeat type of music, mostly instrumental. This hall would more likely resemble a typical mixed-martial arts facility and/or karate dojo and would include

- a few heavy bags of different sizes arranged either in each corner of the facility or in a row;
- a medium-sized ring for sparring practices;

- a TRX-roped gym for body-weight exercises;
- a few different-sized tires for pushing, pulling, and throwing;
- a pair of wing chun punching dummies;
- a pair of BOB punching dummies for self-defense practice and other drills;
- a pair of grappling dummies;
- two to four *makiwara* boards of different thicknesses nailed to walls for hardening the fists;
- at least one wall covered with mirrors for studying one's techniques and movements;
- a matted area for training barefoot.

Yoga Hall—Subtle Armor

This most essential area is accessible to all members interested in deepening their somatic understanding of themselves and thus enhancing the development of their full athletic and human potential.[26] The music played in this studio is mantra music and strictly yoga related. This hall would include

- a nicely matted or carpeted area with a storage for mats,
- pictures of yoga masters in the lineage on walls and other pictures depicting related motifs,

---

[26] A deeper understanding of the vehicle of the body.

- climbing ladders attached to at least one wall to facilitate certain yoga poses,
- a podium or altar where incense or colored lamps can be placed for enhancing the mood of the meditations.

Harmonious Gymnasium Arrangement

A fitness gym that addresses the above needs of a combat athlete would support the warrior's development and expansion of his/her Prana instead of abusing it. To meet that bona fide goal, we offer a unique blend of strength, cardiovascular, and yoga training. We also address one's nutritional needs as based on the Body Type Assessment and offer Ayurvedic-Lifestyle coaching to support the five types of Chi.

When a potential student walks into our gym, he/she is first offered the Ayurvedic Constitution Analysis so that the teacher/coach/trainer learns about their life and current state of health as well as their innate levels of energies. Only then is the proper workout plan recommended. At that point, the student can decide whether they would like to exercise/practice according to the Ayurvedic guidelines obtained from the test, or engage in more conventional training practices, which remain an option.

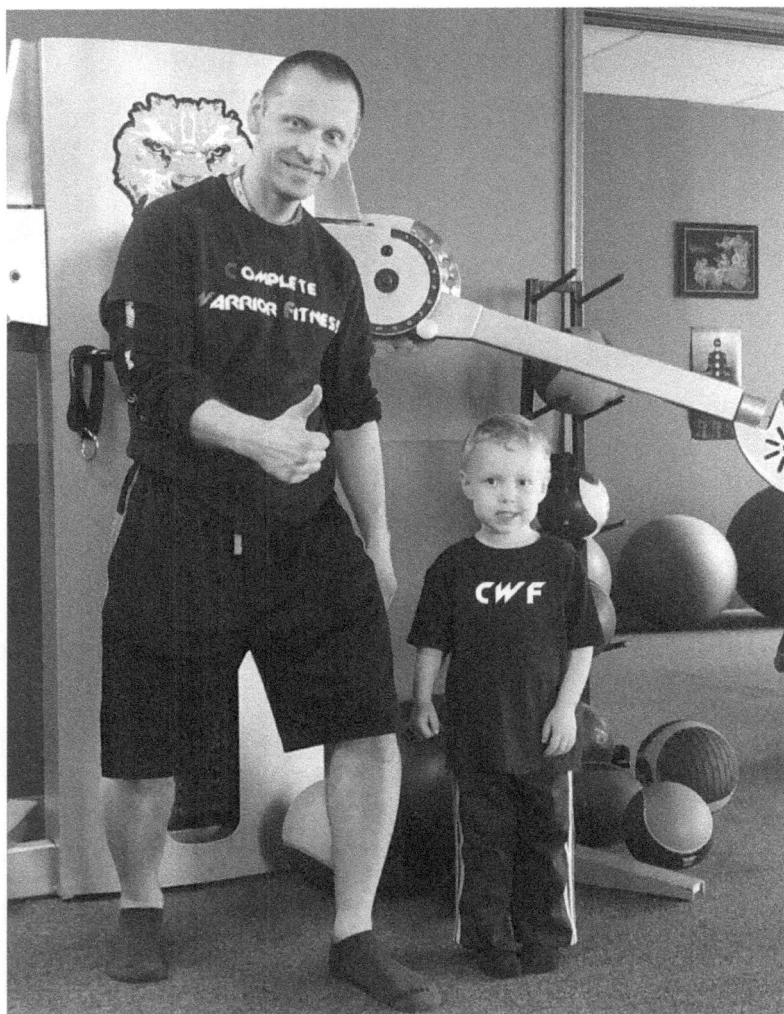

Conclusion

After reading this manual, many of you will have different thoughts. They can all be valid depending on the level of your inner strategy and sophistication in regard to martial arts. As Lao Tsu notes,

The wise student hears of the Tao and practices it diligently.
The average student hears of the Tao and gives it a thought
now and again.
The foolish student hears of the Tao and laughs aloud.
If there were no laughter, the Tao would not be what it is. (41)

However, I believe martial artists can contribute more to the world today with their character and way of action. We are worth more than being fighting experts in the ring or elsewhere. There is already enough aggression in thought, word, and deed that precipitates crime in the world. We will not impress the world by teaching it more about the technical skill of fighting. But we can show the world that true martial artists have a way of life that is harmonious and loving of all creatures under the sun. We can teach more people than just the students who take classes at our dojo. We must reach out, for it is a crucial time…

Some of us are experienced in the practice of martial arts and its philosophy, several of us are quite new to it, and yet some of us are somewhere in the middle. We can all grow more by adding from *Smart Chi* what serves us best to serve the world. We should not be either afraid or lazy to change when the change can benefit us, our families, our students, and the world. As with any endeavor that goes a little out of our comfort zone, the risk is only superficial. Bruce Lee often quoted the Taoist principle "flowing water never goes stale." Thus, in any endeavor, we are wise not to be limited by our present knowledge, not to let it entrap us, and not to cease deepening our perception of life. We should become receptive to the new.

Although it is said, "The easy way seems hard. The highest virtue seems empty…. Real virtue seems unreal," it is also stated at the end that "the Tao alone nourishes and brings everything to fulfillment" (41).

Appendix I

Surrender to Triumph:

The Bhagavad-Gita's Approach to Managing Society

Honorable members of the assembly, dear fellow citizens, the time has come to adopt a completely new and fresh view of our existence. We have given the outdated system a sufficient chance. In fact, a system is judged by its results. We are in a perfect position to begin anew, leaving the past behind and looking into the future with faith grounded in the sound structure that Lord Krishna gave to his warrior-friend Arjuna in these words:

> *"A person in full consciousness of me, knowing me to be the ultimate beneficiary of all sacrifices and austerities, the Supreme Lord of all planets and demigods, and the benefactor and well-wisher of all living entities, attains peace from the pangs of material miseries." (Bg. 5.29)*

Friends, the strategy for peace and happiness on Earth is to follow the all-inclusive and eternal system of bhakti yoga (yoga of devotional service) as described in the ancient treatise known as the *Bhagavad-Gita* (the *Song of God*).

> *"This supreme science was thus received through the chain of disciplic succession, and the saintly kings understood it in that way." (Bg. 4.2)*

The principles of bhakti yoga are based on the spiritual science of the self that Lord Krishna gave to Prince Arjuna 5,000 years ago.

The conversation between Lord Krishna and Arjuna recorded in the *Bhagavad-Gita* is one of the greatest philosophical and religious dialogues ever known. According to a lineage of ancient sages, it is spoken by the Supreme Lord himself:

> *"You are the Supreme Personality of Godhead, the ultimate abode, the purest, the Absolute Truth. You are the eternal, transcendental, original person, the unborn, the greatest. All the great sages such as Narada, Asita, Devala, and Vyasa confirm this truth about you, and now you yourself are declaring it to me." (Bg. 10.12–13)*

The pillars of spirituality are now almost completely misunderstood and forgotten. The situation is becoming worse in the world, and people are calling out for real protection from the miseries that assail them from the misdirected leaders. We are trying to rule human society, but because we lack spiritual knowledge, we are in a chaotic condition. The plan presented here by me is called the Threefold Luminous Pillar Approach (TLPA).[27] It expands and elaborates on the verse from the first paragraph of this chapter, Bg. 5.29. The transitional method, or the Bridging Method, is added to the TLPA to accommodate everyone, as is a list of Four Rare Benefits that our society will acquire by following the TLPA.

Lastly, in our endeavor to introduce the TLPA in society's educational institutions, we should augment it by a more elaborate explanation of the teachings of the *Bhagavad-Gita*, of which a succinct summary is included. And now, if you kindly allow me, I am prepared to present Lord Krishna's plan to eliminate the obstinate elements in our society.

Three-fold Luminous Pillar Approach

The perfection of consciousness is given by Lord Krishna to the warrior Arjuna in these words:

> *"Engage your mind always in thinking of me, become my devotee, offer obeisances to me, and worship me. Being completely absorbed in me, surely you will come to me." (Bg. 9.34)*

---

[27] The idea has been adapted by the author from his own *Transcendental Warrior* book trilogy (Vol. II).

This state of consciousness is an advanced one and is usually attained after practicing the following method for some time:

> *"My dear Arjuna, O winner of wealth, if you cannot fix your mind upon me without deviation, then follow the regulative principles of bhakti-yoga. In this way develop a desire to attain me."* (Bg. 12.9)

The principles of bhakti yoga include the introduction of positive activities, the Three Luminous pillars, and the gradual, yet automatic, removal of detrimental activities described below as the Dark Pillars. By engaging in the practices of bhakti-yoga, non-healthy behavior is naturally dissipated, just as is darkness when the light is turned on.

1st LUMINOUS PILLAR.
The Method of Offering.

The method of offering dissipates or neutralizes the two dark pillars of meat-eating and illicit sexual relations.

Because both meat-eating and illicit sex are the culmination of selfish exploitation stemming from a taking nature rather than a giving one, learning how to offer one's things, one's works and even one's very self, naturally removes the hard-heartedness and ego-centricity necessary to be involved in animal slaughter and illicit sex. As long as we inflict unnecessary pain on other living entities, we will find ourselves unable to access the fully developed sense of mercy and compassion. Srila Prabhupada states that "every living creature is a son of the Supreme Lord, and He does not tolerate even an ant's being killed. One has to pay for it. So indulgence in animal killing for the taste of the tongue is the grossest kind of ignorance. A human being has no need to kill animals, because God has provided so many nice things." (Bg. 14.16, purport) He further elaborates: "The maintenance of slaughterhouses for the satisfaction of the tongue and the killing of animals unnecessarily should never be sanctioned by a government.... According to the law of necessity, first of all human society must try to produce grains and vegetables, but if they fail in this, they can indulge in flesh eating.... The conclusion is that the earth produces sufficient grain to feed the entire population, but the distribution of this grain is restricted due to trade regulations and a desire for profit."

> "If one offers me with love and devotion a leaf, a flower, fruit, or water, I will accept it." (Bg. 9.16)

Srila Prabhupada explains about the verse above that "one who loves Krishna will give him whatever he wants, and avoid offering anything which is undesirable or unasked. If he desired such things as offerings, he would have said so.... Vegetables, grains, fruits, milk, and water are the proper foods for human beings and are prescribed by Lord Krishna himself." (Bg. 9.26, purport) Sexual activities outside of marriage or sexual activities not meant to create progeny, destroys our external (body) and internal (heart and mind) quality of cleanliness. Srila Prabhupada cautions us in the following words: "The highest pleasure in terms of matter is sex pleasure. The whole world is moving under its spell, and a materialist cannot work at all without this motivation. But a person engaged in Krishna consciousness can work with greater vigor without sex pleasure, which he avoids. That is the test in spiritual realization." (Bg. 5.21, purport)

Lord Krishna states in the *Bhagavad-Gita*,

> "I am the strength of the strong, devoid of passion and desire. I am sex life which is not contrary to religious principles." (Bg. 7.11)

Srila Prabhupada elucidates that "one should always remember that the genitals, sexual pleasure, the woman, and the offspring are all related in the service of the Lord, and one who forgets this relationship in the service of the Supreme Lord becomes subjected to...miseries of material existence." (SB 2.10.26, purport) It is recommended that one is married to one woman and uses one's sexual potency to help other living entities to come into this world. Enjoying sex is natural, especially if it leads to pregnancy and to properly raised children. When we use sex like this, it becomes our offering to Lord Krishna. It is the responsibility of each warrior to raise powerful warrior children so that we can all enter the Golden Age as predicted in the scriptures.

2nd LUMINOUS PILLAR.
The Method of Hearing.

The method of hearing disspates or neutralizes the third dark pillar of intoxication.

When we indulge in alcohol, drugs, tobacco, or even caffeinated products, our vision becomes distorted, and we lose clarity of thinking and the ability to live simply. The quality of austerity, or not engaging in unnecessary sense pleasure, is further undermined. Intoxication causes us to forget about Lord Krishna. Without proper remembrance of Lord Krishna, our actions will be incited by selfish desires rather than his will. How can we lead our society if our government officials take intoxicants? Srila Prabhupada clarifies:

> *"Being distressed by their circumstances, they [people] take shelter of intoxication, and thus they*

> *sink further into ignorance. Their future is very*
> *dark." (Bg. 14.17, purport)*

Material distress, which leads to material intoxication as a cure, can immediately be mitigated by hearing, because through hearing from a perfected source we gain knowledge and remembrance of our enduring self.

Lord Krishnsa provided and directed us to use his royal intoxicant known as his holy name: "Always chanting my glories, endeavoring with great determination, bowing down before me, these great souls perpetually worship me with devotion," (Bg. 9.14) and "of vibrations I am the transcendental Om. Of sacrifices I am the chanting of the holy names [japa], and of immovable things, I am the Himalayas." (Bg. 10.25) In the purport to the latter verse, Srila Prabhupada tells us, "Of all sacrifices, the chanting of Hare Krishna, Hare Krishna, Krishna Krishna, Hare Hare, Hare Rama, Hare Rama, Rama Rama, Hare Hare is the purest representation of Krishna, [because] there is no question of violence. It is the simplest and the purest."

The hearing of the holy name makes us remember the Lord and makes his presence more perceptible to us. The royal intoxicant is described in these words: "I do not know how much nectar the two syllables 'Krish-na' have produced. When the holy name of Krishna is chanted, it appears to dance within the mouth. We then desire many, many mouths. When the name enters the holes of the ears, we desire many millions of ears. And when the holy name dances in the courtyard of the heart, it conquers the activities of the mind, and therefore all the senses become inert [from spiritual ecstasy]." (Rupa Goswami, as quoted by Prabhupada, Cc., Antya, 1.9 purport) Invite your family and friends to chant the holy name with you (use musical instruments as well). Throw a holy name party at your home and intoxicate yourself royally.

3rd LUMINOUS PILLAR.
The Method of Detachment.

The method of detachment dissipates or neutralizes the dark pillar of gambling.

Externally, gambling comes in the form of lottery cards, casinos, and speculative business ventures. Internally, gambling comes as speculating about the nature of spirituality while relying solely on our own intelligence. Basically, a gambler makes an attempt to gain much with little effort, but the results are highly unpredictable. We gamble when we search whimsically to enjoy and then try to justify our actions by inventing spiritual or moral principles that appeal to us. We waste our time and endanger our spiritual consciousness when we gamble.

Gambling brings on the tendency to see things unequally—in terms of gain and loss and not in terms of Lord Krishna's satisfaction. Risking what you honestly earned for quick gain and entertainment destroys the motivation to work sincerely for Krishna. Thus, the quality of truthfulness is undermined. By developing detachment, the insatiable need to have more for less, to cheat the system, our friends, our family, our selves, is naturally vanquished, allowing truthfulness to flourish.

Lord Krishna reveals more to Arjuna in response to his doubts about following the process:

> *"O mighty-armed son of Kunti, it is undoubtedly very difficult to curb the restless mind, but it is possible by suitable practice [bhakti yoga] and by detachment." (Bg. 6.34)*

As we guide our families and society to peace and prosperity, we should always see that our dependants avoid gambling while sincerely following the other principles such as chanting the holy name of Krishna.

Srila Prabhupada enlightens us: "Attachment for sense enjoyment...is very strong. Therefore, one must learn detachment by discussion of spiritual science based on authoritative scriptures, and one must hear from persons who are actually in knowledge." (Bg. 15.3, purport) This honest approach to spiritual practice will ensure victory in other realms of action when taking calculated risks for Lord Krishna's sake becomes necessary. In the words of Sanjaya,

"Wherever there is Krishna, the master of all mystics, and wherever there is Arjuna [his friend and servant], the supreme archer, there will also certainly be opulence, victory, extraordinary power, and morality." (Bg. 18.78)

When one has no desire to follow the regulative principles of bhakti yoga, then one can still surrender one's work to Lord Krishna (Bg. 12.10) and use the Bridging Method: [28]

"Whatever you do, whatever you eat, whatever you offer or give away, and whatever austerities you perform—do that, O son of Kunti, as an offering to me." (Bg. 9.27)

And for those attached to work, the person should try to give up the results, or part of the results, of his/her work for Lord Krishna.

If, however, one thinks that is still not possible, Lord Krishna extends the bridge even further:

"Then try to act giving up all results of your work...for by such renunciation one can attain peace of mind." (Bg. 12.11–12)

Such sacrifice of one's work to a good cause (charity, social service, sacrifice for one's country, etc.) will gradually make

---

[28] One is not allowed to intentionally offer the sinful activities discussed here.

one ready to follow the aforementioned principles and advance on the path to completely purify one's character for the Lord's glory.

Four Rare Benefits

Dear leaders, by sincerely and determinedly following the teachings of the *Bhagavad-Gita*, our dependents will acquire the Four Rare Benefits: (Prabhupada, *Nectar of Devotion*, 3)

1. Immediate relief from all kinds of material distress (both by internal transformation and by actually affecting the external environment as stated in the verse). (Bg. 5.29)
2. All-auspiciousness (by fully reawakening divine qualities of character mentioned above, such as compassion, cleanliness, etc., we positively influence everyone and everything around us).
3. Enjoyment of spiritual (transcendental) pleasure.
4. The ability to attract the protection and love of Lord Krishna. We will revive our dormant relationship with him. "But whoever renders service unto me in devotion is a friend, is in me, and I am also a friend to him." (Bg. 9.29)

In due course of time, as the *Bhagavad-Gita's* principles are taught and implemented in detail in schools, the social consciousness will change, everyone will become satisfied and happy, and the results will be magnificent. The following four verses of the *Bhagavad-Gita* summarize its entire teachings:

> *"I am the source of all spiritual and material worlds. Everything emanates from me. The wise who perfectly know this engage in my devotional service and worship me with all their hearts." (Bg. 10.8)*

In the above verse, Lord Krishna sums up his opulences and how one acts upon realizing this truth.

> *"The thoughts of my pure devotees dwell in me, their lives are fully devoted to my service, and they derive great satisfaction and bliss from always enlightening one another and conversing about me." (Bg. 10.9)*

Lord Krishna explains in the verse above how his pure servant worships him.

> *"To those who are constantly devoted to serving me with love, I give the understanding by which they can come to me." (Bg. 10.10)*

Above and in the next verse, the Lord gives us an idea of the reciprocation that takes place between him and the pure servant.

"To show them special mercy, I, dwelling in their hearts, destroy with the shining lamp of knowledge the darkness born of ignorance." (Bg. 10.11)

As our leaders educate their dependents about this, the citizens will come to the standard. In the words of Srila Prabhupada, "It is the duty of everyone to mold his life in such a way that he will not forget Krishna in any circumstance." (Bg. 9.27, purport) Those who rule should first follow the principles and see that the subjects get inspired by their example to receive such an education.

"Whatever action a great man performs, common men follow. And whatever standards he sets by exemplary acts, all the world pursues." (Bg. 3.21)

My friends, Lord Krishna recommends for us to live in the highest consciousness while managing our affairs on Earth and guarantees the results we have discussed. The Threefold Luminous Pillar Approach introduces practical tenets of bhakti yoga while gradually removing behavioral patterns detrimental to our prosperous future. Therefore, it behooves us to first understand it and then implement accordingly. Let us give ourselves a chance to become part of Lord Krishna's eternal standard and triumph over all difficulties. Thank you for your attention.

Appendix II

The Importance of Nutrition in the Mode of Goodness

As you may recall, the three modes of nature exist not only in nature but also in human beings. Thus, some of us are predominantly affected by the mode of goodness; some, passion; and some, ignorance. The mental constitution analysis in chapter II evaluates that. It is possible to consume foods that are in the mode of goodness and thus facilitate—along with proper training, breathing, mantra—the transferring of our consciousness to the mode of goodness. Staying in the mode of goodness ensures that we do not abuse or misuse our martial capacity. On top of that, it will quicken our evolution on the yoga ladder and allow us to ascend to samadhi, the topmost rung of yoga.

Human beings, especially those involved in physical training, are most suited to a vegetarian diet, which is closer to the mode of goodness. Over the years, there has been a rise of vegetarian and vegan athletes all over the world. We may mention such names as Carl Lewis (Olympic runner), Surya Bonaly (Olympic figure skater), Roger Brown (professional football player), Peter Burwash (tennis pro), Chris Campbell (Olympic medalist in wrestling), Murray Rose (Olympic gold medalist in swimming), Dave Scott (six-time Ironman Triathlon winner). Even my karate teacher, a high-ranking karateka, is a vegetarian.

First of all, human beings can survive on meat, but they are not biologically made for it. Take human teeth, for instance. They are like those of plant-eating animals, suited to grinding and chewing rather than ripping and tearing. Carnivorous animals usually tear the prey apart and swallow chunks of flesh without chewing them. Therefore, they do not possess molars. Neither are their jaws capable of moving sideways in a chewing motion. Also, human hands are not equipped with sharp claws but instead have the opposable thumb needed for those who harvest their food. (Prabhupada, *Higher Taste*, 1)

Meat requires strong digestive juices if it is not to rot in the stomach. Humans and other plant-eating animals produce acid one-twentieth the strength of the stomach acids found in carnivores. Carnivores also have a relatively short intestinal tract; meat rots quickly and must be moved through the body before it becomes toxic to the eater. Carnivores possess alimentary canals only three times the length of their bodies. Humans and other plant-eaters have alimentary canals twelve times their body length. As a result, the bodies of humans who do consume meat are stressed by having to move it through such long intestines. The toxins produced tend to alter their natural metabolism, which is made for the digestion of carbohydrates. Furthermore, so much extra energy going into digestion tends to divert life energy from other functions, including thinking. Meat consumption means that you absorb many toxic wastes that would otherwise be expelled from the animal's body as urine. (3)

The kidneys are responsible for the elimination of toxins. Meat eaters strain their kidneys, overloading them daily with substances produced during the body's attempt to digest meat. The kidneys of even moderate meat-eaters have to do three times more work than the kidneys of their vegetarian counterparts. While you are young, you can no doubt cope with the added stress, but as you age, the risk of kidney disease and renal failure increases. (3)

Meat-eating humans also struggle to deal with excessive animal fats. Natural carnivores can metabolize almost unlimited amounts of cholesterol and fat without negative effect, but humans cannot. Over a period of years, an excess of uneliminated fats builds up, arteries harden, and stroke or heart attack become imminent. (3–4)

There is also a higher chance of contracting colon cancer among meat-eaters, again, because of the toxic wastes moved to the digestive system after initial digestion in the stomach. Aside from that, meat of industrially raised animals contains preservatives, antibiotics, and the remains of untreated animal diseases. Meat is often loaded with

DDT, arsenic (used in cattle food as a growth stimulant), sodium sulfate (which gives meat a "fresh" red color), and DES (a synthetic hormone that increases a chance of cancer). (9)

For many people, the single-most compelling evidence against meat-eating is the well-documented correlation between meat consumption and heart disease. America has the highest rate of meat consumption in the world, and in America, one out of every two persons will die of heart-related complications. Such diseases are lower in nations where meat consumption is low. (10)

What about the need for dietary protein? Many powerful animals get their protein from vegetable sources—think of elephants, bulls, and rhinoceroses. Each of these animals is both powerful and vegetarian. Flesh foods do not contain any amino acids that cannot be obtained from plant foods eaten in a proper combination. The famous bodybuilder Bill Pearl confirms,

> *You do not need meat for protein. About half of the world population does not eat meat for religious or other reasons. There are also large groups of people in the United States, such as the Seventh Day Adventists, who do not eat meat at all—and display much better health than the average American.... Where do they obtain their protein? The answer is simple: proteins are a part of virtually every natural food available to man. Every plant, every seed, and every fruit contains*

some protein. It is virtually impossible not to obtain enough protein on any diet of natural foods. The long-held belief that meat proteins are superior to vegetable proteins has been disapproved. Recent research has demonstrated that animal proteins in any amounts have a detrimental effect on health and that vegetable proteins, formerly believed to be incomplete or inferior to animal proteins, are actually biologically as good or better than animal proteins.... You also do not need meat protein for strength. (Pearl, 34)

The idea that large amounts of protein are required for energy and strength is a myth. When proteins are digested, they break down into amino acids, which the body uses for growth and tissue replacement. The body itself can synthesize all but eight of the twenty-two amino acids. Those eight essential amino acids are found in abundance in non-flesh foods. (*Higher Taste*, 10)

When we consume foods from the plant kingdom, we combine our assimilation of amino acids with the assimilation of other essential nutrients for proper anabolism (tissue growth), such as carbohydrates, vitamins, minerals, enzymes, hormones, chlorophyll, etc. Besides, the body uses protein as a last resort; when we don't consume enough carbohydrates, the body will use protein for energy. The body's main source of energy comes from carbohydrates. When we eat too much protein, the body's energy capacity is reduced. Physical tests show that vegetarians are able to perform physical tasks two to three times longer than meat-eaters before exhaustion sets in. They also fully recover from fatigue up to five times faster. (Rosen, 5–6)

Some people may already know that the current position of the American Dietetic Association recommends a meatless diet as healthier and adequate when appropriately planned. Also, the *Dietary Guidelines for Americans* issued by the US Department of Agriculture and US Department of Health and Human Services represents the federal policy on the role of dietary factors in health and disease prevention: "Vegetarian diets are consistent with the Dietary Guidelines and can meet Recommended Dietary Allowances for nutrients. Protein is not limiting in vegetarian diets as long as the variety and amounts of foods consumed are adequate." (7)

From the point of view of ethics, a true human being, a gentleman or gentlewoman, does not wish to cause undue suffering to any living entity. Slaughtering an animal is painful for the animal and causes its suffering. On the physical and emotional levels, both animals and humans are feeling creatures. Irrespective of whether we kill them slowly or quickly, the animals suffer. We are each given a material body and a lifespan. To cut another entity's lifespan short without good cause is unethical or, some may say, sinful.

The majority of biologists consider consciousness only in terms of behavior. They do not look at behavior as a symptom of a spiritual presence in the entity. This is called material reductionism. Many biologists and other such scientists do not consider animals sentient. That is, there is no real difference between stones and dogs. Whatever sensation an animal experiences can never be compared to the human experience. Scientists use this argument to justify laboratory experiments on animals, as well as for meat-eating.

However, this argument cannot stand up to reason. If we examine animals, we will see that they are characterized by all the same traits as humans. That is how we determine that they are alive. Why do animals being led to slaughter struggle? Stones do not struggle when they are being brought to destruction, because they are not alive. What is the difference between stones (or dead bodies) and living entities? Animals eat and people eat; animals sleep and people sleep; animals bleed and people bleed; animals reproduce and people reproduce. Similarly, both animals and humans experience pain and pleasure. Can we place a value on the actual degree of an animal's suffering when compared to a human's? That doesn't seem logical.

Because our society has learned to devalue animal suffering, it does not use anesthetics to ease the pain animals may feel. Cruelty is common in stockyards. Sick and injured animals may live for days before being slaughtered. Factory farming is horrendously cruel. In factory henhouses, a number of hens are raised in 12-by-18-inch cages. The hens are driven mad by the lack of space, and they attempt to peck each other to death.

Farmers then de-beak the birds, a painful process in itself. Then hens are kept as long as they lay a certain number of eggs in a week. If they fail to meet their quota, they are culled and slaughtered.

Although most eggs go unfertilized, roosters are allowed to fertilize a certain number of eggs to keep up the production of hens. Male chicks are disposed of at hatching by "chick-pullers." Up to 500,000 male chicks are born in the U.S. daily. They are culled from the females and then placed in plastic bags, where they often suffocate or are crushed under other chicks. Some remain alive long enough to be ground up as livestock feed or fertilizer.

Most countries have inhumane laws regarding animal slaughter. Those who are interested should inform themselves of these laws. Animal killing, regardless of the animal's level of development, breeds callousness, insensitivity toward other beings, and sadism, and it proves a lack of reverence for life.

Another point to consider is the impact your diet has on economy. From the economic vantage point, consider the following statistics: one acre of wheat yields 353 pounds of protein, one acre of corn yields 286 pounds of protein, and one acre of rice yields 542 pounds of protein. Feed protein conversion efficiency of cattle is about 6 percent. This means that one acre of corn used to raise a steer will yield only 17 pounds of beef protein.

It has been estimated that raising livestock consumes eight times more water than growing vegetables or grains because the cattle drink and the crops that feed them must also be watered. (8) Another piece of evidence is that meat consumption produces methane, which is one of the four greenhouse gases contributing to global warming. For example, the 1.3 billion cattle in the world produce one-fifth of all the methane emitted in the atmosphere. Most people are aware that the world's priceless rainforests are being destroyed day by day as the lumber and meat industries transform them into giant pastures to provide cheap beef. (8)

Last but not least is the aesthetic factor. Most of us are aware that the odor of animal and fish carcasses is horrible and is tolerated only with the help of intoxication to dull the senses. People often dress meat with spices and sauces, and cook it so that it is finally accepted by the body without repulsion. Most of us would not dare to eat raw meat, what to speak of personally slaughtering an animal. Most children have to be forced to eat the first portions of a fish. On the other hand, dishes prepared from the plant kingdom are colorful and pleasing to the eye, the nose, and the tongue.

Bibliography

Berkovich–Ohana, Aviva, Meytal Wilf, Roni Kahana, Amos Arieli, and Rafael Malach. "Repetitive Speech Elicits Widespread Deactivation in the Human Cortex: The 'Mantra' Effect?" *Brain and Behavior* 5, no. 7 (July 2015). https://doi.org/10.1002/brb3.346.

Epel, Elissa, Jennifer Daubenmier, Judith T. Moskowitz, Susan Folkman, and Elizabeth Blackburn. "Can Meditation Slow Rate of Cellular Aging? Cognitive Stress, Mindfulness, and Telomeres." *Annals of the New York Academy of Sciences* 1172, no. 1 (August 2009): 34–53. https://doi.org/10.1111/j.1749-6632.2009.04414.x.

Frawley, David. *Ayurveda and the Mind: The Healing of Consciousness.* Twin Lakes, Wisconsin: Lotus Press, 2007.

———. *Yoga and Ayurveda: Self-Healing and Self-Realization.* Twin Lakes, Wisconsin: Lotus Press, 1999.

Frawley, David, and Sandra Summerfield Kozak. *Yoga for Your Type: An Ayurvedic Approach to Your Asana Practice.* Twin Lakes, Wisconsin: Lotus Press, 2009.

Frawley, David, and Vasant Lad. *The Yoga of Herbs: An Ayurvedic Guide to Herbal Medicine.* Twin Lakes, Wisconsin: Lotus Press, 1988

Frawley, David, and Subhash Ranade. *Ayurveda, Nature's Medicine.* Twin Lakes, Wisconsin: Lotus Press, 2001.

Frawley, David, Subhash Ranade, and Avinash Lele. *Ayurveda and*

Marma Therapy: Energy Points in Yogic Healing. Twin Lakes, Wisconsin: Lotus Press, 2012.

Gastelu, Daniel, and Frederick Hatfield. *Specialist in Performance Nutrition: The Complete Guide.* Carpinteria, California: International Sports Sciences Association, 2000.

Lad, Vasant. *The Complete Book of Ayurvedic Home Remedies.* New York: Harmony Books, 1998.

Oyama, Mas. *Mas Oyama's Complete Karate Course.* New York: Sterling, 1998.

Pearl, Bill. *Bill Pearl's Keys to the Inner Universe.* Edited by Leroy R. Perry Jr. Phoenix, Oregon: Bill Pearl Enterprises, 2000.

Prabhupada, A. C. Bhaktivedanta Swami. *Bhagavad-Gita As It Is.* Victoria, Australia: Bhaktivedanta Book Trust, 1994.
———. *The Higher Taste.* Los Angeles: Bhaktivedanta Book Trust, 1991.

———. *Sri Chaitanya-charitamrita.* Australia: Bhaktivedanta Book Trust, 1996.

———. *Srimad Bhagavatam.* Los Angeles: Bhaktivedanta Book Trust, 1987.

Rosen, Steven. *Diet for Transcendence: Vegetarianism and the World Religions.* Badger, CA: Torchlight Publishing, 1997.

Sheldon, William H., Stanley S. Stevens, and William B. Tucker. *The Varieties of Human Physique: An Introduction to Constitutional Psychology.* New York: Harper & Brothers, 1940.

Svoboda, Robert E. *Prakriti: Your Ayurvedic Constitution,* 2nd ed. Bellingham, Washington: Sadhana Publications, 1998.

Tiwari, Maya. *A Life of Balance: The Complete Guide to Ayurvedic Nutrition and Body Types with Recipes*. Rochester, Vermont: Healing Arts Press, 1995.

Tsu, Lao. *Tao Te Ching*, 25th anniversary ed. Translated by Gia-Fu Feng and Jane English. New York: Vintage Books, 1997.
Watson, George. *Nutrition and Your Mind: The Psychochemical Response*. New York: Harper & Row, 1972.

Whitaker, Justin. "The Effectiveness of Meditation: A Meta-Analysis." *American Buddhist Perspectives* (blog). *Patheos*, January 12, 2014, http://www.patheos.com/blogs/americanbuddhist/2014/01/the-effectiveness-of-meditation-a-meta-analysis.html.

Xu, Jian, Alexandra Vik, Inge R. Groote, Jim Lagopoulos, Are Holen, Oyvind Ellingsen, Asta K. Haberg, et al. "Nondirective Meditation Activates Default Mode Network and Areas Associated with Memory Retrieval and Emotional Processing." *Frontiers in Human Neuroscience* 8, no. 86 (February 2014). https://doi.org/10.3389/fnhum.2014.00086.

Index

About the Author

A disciple of His Holiness Chandramauli Swami who comes in the line of bhakti yogis, and a graduate student of American Institute of Vedic Studies under the auspices of Vamadeva Shastri (Dr. David Frawley), Arkadiusz Madej, a.k.a. Arjunacharya Dasa, has come a long way to present this work.

Arjunacharya is an International Sports Sciences Association Master Trainer and Ayurvedic Lifestyle Consultant who has been an avid practitioner of karate throughout his life. Arjunacharya's approach to coaching has a multidimensional basis that integrates three essential aspects of human health: the physical, emotional, and spiritual. It aims at providing everyone with knowledge on how to lead a balanced, dynamic, and satisfying lifestyle. Such an approach further combines the latest discoveries in the fields of fitness and science with the ancient and well-proven principles found in the medical books of India. Arjunacharya's clients are offered a methodology for genuine fitness to "feel the power!" as he says.

As an Elmhurst College honors graduate in liberal arts with a major in philosophy and minor in psychology, Ark loves writing, educating, and sharing his knowledge and practical realization. He is currently pursuing his doctoral studies in the field of natural medicine.

In 2005, he authored a complete exposition of his vision of life in the *Transcendental Warrior* trilogy. In 2010, he released *Krishna Warrior Fitness Challenge*, a book on functional fitness with an accompanying demo DVD. The book you are holding in your hands, which uniquely combines practical knowledge of Ayurveda, fitness training, and martial arts, comes as no surprise and presents no ordinary knowledge.

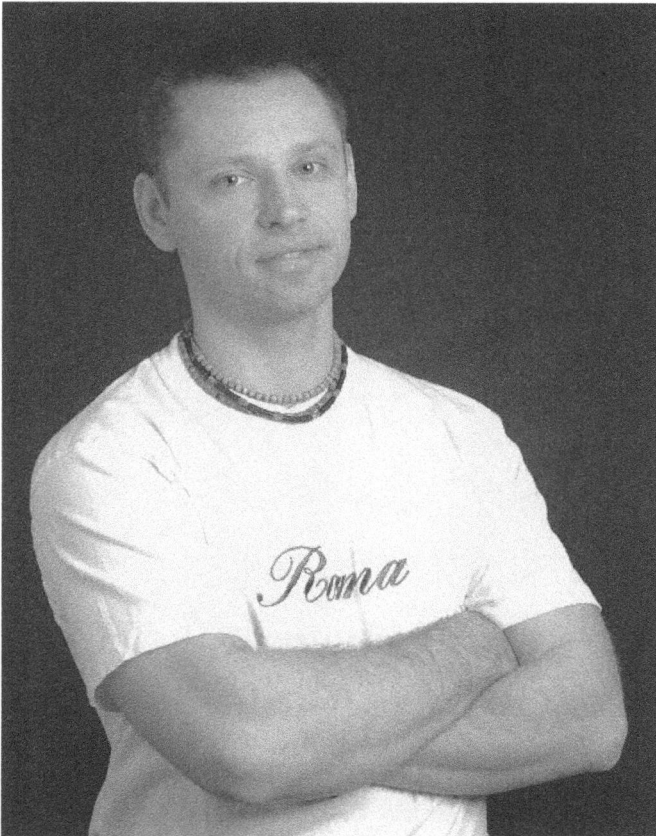